CREATE A YOGA PRACTICE FOR KIDS
FUN, FLEXIBILITY, AND FOCUS

Praise for *Create a Yoga Practice for Kids*

"Most of the yogis who attend our yoga studio have children and are always looking for ways to interest their children in yoga. While we offer Family Yoga and Kids Yoga, the demand for "more for the children" continues. This book offers parents and yoga teachers a way to easily introduce yoga into the lives of our children, and it does so in a presentation that is at once simple, fun, and delightful! I am confident this book will be on my shelves at the studio, so that when parents clamor for more kids yoga, I can recommend this book!"

> —**D'ana Baptiste,** co-creator of the Baptiste Power Yoga Institute and
> Director of D'ana Baptiste Studios.

"It feels like the authors have emptied their hearts to share the beauty of yoga with children, teachers, and parents. There is so much richness in the book. The relaxation techniques at the end of the book are amazing. One of my 11 year old students said the other day, "I love Yoga because it begins with you are beautiful and perfect not that you are bad and wrong." My heart dances when people like Yael and Matthew take their time and energy to serve children and graciously and generously share so much."

> —**Sheryl Edsall**, Director of Naturally Yoga in New Jersey
> and creator of Barefoot Kids Yoga.

"Your book is a wonderful gift to children, teachers, and families. As a parent of four young children and as a clinical social worker, I see a desperate need for *Create a Yoga Practice for Kids*. In this very fast paced world, the book offers a simple and creative way for teachers and families to connect with children, while encouraging exercise and relaxation. It gives children skills that will nurture them through their entire lives."

> —**Elizabeth Q. Finlinson**, L.C.S.W., Salt Lake City, Utah.

"Fun, Flexibility and Focus are just three of the many great benefits that can come from sharing a Yoga Practice with children. This book gives very clear, easy to follow instructions and suggestions to help any teacher, parent or friend begin a regular and successful Yoga Practice with children of all ages. The more children experience Peace, Joy, Health and Happiness the less Dis-ease and Dis-harmony we will have in the world. Drops make Oceans. Thank you, Yael and Matthew, for contributing to the Ocean of Peace."

> Om Shanti.
> —**Satya Greenstone**, Integral Yoga Teacher Training, Satchidananda
> AshramYogaville, Virginia.

CREATE A YOGA PRACTICE
FOR KIDS

FUN, FLEXIBILITY, AND FOCUS

By
Yael Calhoun
and
Matthew R. Calhoun

Illustrated by Carol Anne Coogan

SUNSTONE PRESS

SANTA FE

Sunstone books may be purchased for educational, business, or sales promotional use. For information please write: Special Markets Department, Sunstone Press, P.O. Box 2321, Santa Fe, New Mexico 87504-2321.

Library of Congress Cataloging-in-Publication Data:

Calhoun, Yael.
    Create a yoga practice for kids : fun, flexibility, and focus / by Yael Calhoun and Matthew R. Calhoun ; illustrated by Carol Anne Coogan.
      p. cm.
    ISBN 0-86534-490-6 (pbk. : alk. paper)
    1. Hatha yoga for children--Handbooks, manuals, etc. 2. Exercise for children--Handbooks, manuals, etc. I. Calhoun, Matthew R. II. Coogan, Carol Anne. III. Title.

RA781.7.C35 2006
613.7'046083--dc22

                                                              2006012829

Published in

WWW.SUNSTONEPRESS.COM
SUNSTONE PRESS / POST OFFICE BOX 2321 / SANTA FE, NM 87504-2321 /USA
(505) 988-4418 / ORDERS ONLY (800) 243-5644 / FAX (505) 988-1025

We would like to extend special thanks to
Lilias Folan for her inspiration and her generosity
of spirit in reviewing our manuscript
and sharing her wisdom.

Be like the bird
Who halting in his flight
On limb too slight
Feels it give way beneath him,
Yet sings
Knowing he hath wings.
—Victor Hugo

To the kids at Granite Elementary who inspired this
book. And to Alex, Sam, and Ben Isaac—who inspire
me each day.
—YC

To my parents, Joy and Ted, who have always
encouraged me to follow my own path.
—MRC

For all children, everywhere. And for all those who
teach, nurture and help children grow.
—CC

Contents

Foreword

*T*here's no substitute for learning something when you're young. What enters into the open, pliable minds of children settles deeply into their cells. What is practiced integrates so profoundly that it weaves into the fabric of their beings. Those habits we cultivate when we are young have great momentum and carry over effortlessly into adulthood. So when Yael asked me what I thought about her writing a book on yoga for children, I answered with a resounding "Yes!"

The downturn in children's fitness levels in the past 10 years is not breaking news. Articles blaming poor diet and sedentary lifestyles for the sudden rise in childhood obesity appear regularly in all manner of periodicals, from mainstream newspapers to specialty magazines. Where children once explored the outdoors for fun, most now spend playtime in the two-dimensional worlds of television and the Internet. As a result, nine million American children—that's 15 percent of kids and teenagers—are obese, triple the total in 1980.

These children not only face the risk of joining the looming diabetes epidemic, but, according to a December 2004 article in Education Weekly, students with health issues are not as capable of learning as are their healthy counterparts. A 2002 study by the California Department of Education presented anecdotal support for this theory. Education Weekly wrote, "Physically fit youngsters in the study posted significantly higher scores on math and reading tests, and those who met minimum fitness levels in three or more areas showed the greatest gains in academic achievement."

At the same time, millions of adults have begun seeking balanced fitness and inner tranquility through the practice of yoga, which is enjoying its largest number of practitioners in history. When I studied yoga at the Ramamani Iyengar Memorial Yoga Institute in Pune, India in 1989, I was inspired to see that the children's classes were packed with eager young yogis—and they were having a great time. Why not let American kids in on the fun?

The physical and physiological benefits alone—toned muscles, upright posture, a balanced nervous system, and free and healthy breathing patterns, among many others—are enough to set a child on a track that will serve her well throughout life. As the physical body comes into balance, the mind follows. Practicing yoga can help a child develop concentration, patience, gentleness, strength, creativity and stability. These are habits we'd all love to cultivate. They are the building blocks that create the foundation for a happy life.

Create a Yoga Practice for Kids presents a fun and engaging way for parents and yoga teachers to introduce kids to the 3,000-year-old practice of yoga. Practice has to be fun, however, to capture a child's fancy. Using imaginative theme practices (with such intriguing titles as "Poses that Melt" and "Poses You can do in Line and those you Cannot!"), poses named for funny and familiar members of the animal kingdom, and mind-melting relaxation exercises, this book encourages physical coordination, relaxation, introspection, laughter and creativity. With its explicit instructions and explanations of the benefits of each pose, it also provides an opportunity for kids and parents to discover yoga together. Enjoy this book!

—Charlotte Bell
Salt Lake City, Utah

Charlotte Bell has taught yoga and meditation since 1986. Based in Salt Lake City, she teaches workshops, retreats, teacher trainings and yoga river trips throughout the intermountain West and Canada.

Preface

I am a long-time yoga practitioner, teacher, and mom. The idea for this book came to me as I was teaching yoga at my kids' elementary school. Several students asked for copies of that day's practice so they could do it at home. Parents also have asked me for copies of our Final Relaxation to do before bed with their kids. Such kid comments as: "I really needed this"; "Oh, I love this part;" "Promise you won't start until I get back from the bathroom;" and, "I feel so relaxed now," have reinforced my feeling that kids appreciate an integrated sequencing of poses that celebrates yoga's benefits and beauty.

Most of my teaching career has been spent teaching elementary school. I bring this classroom experience to my yoga teaching: how to offer a complete lesson that flows and how to keep students actively involved in their own learning. I have taught kids' yoga in a variety of settings, including a boys' and girls' club, an elementary school, a camp for the disabled, and a YWCA shelter. I also teach adult yoga.

Creating an opportunity for kids to get excited about yoga and perhaps offering them a life-long tool for physical and emotional health is the reason for this book.

Namaste.

—Yael Calhoun
Sandy, Utah

Many years ago, when I was an undergrad at the high-stress University of Chicago, I was visiting home for the weekend. My mother, Joy, suggested that I check out a yoga program on public television. She said that yoga would serve as a shield for me in life. I turned on *Lilias, Yoga and You!* and began to follow Lilias Folan's words. During a "Sponge" relaxation, she suggested that I put my problems aside for now, and not to worry, because they would still be there later. At this unexpected suggestion, my whole body and spirit relaxed in such a delightful way, I felt I was floating. Although she never met me, Lilias became my teacher through her TV shows, books, and videos. She had the magical quality of making me feel she was in the room with me, speaking to me directly.

In my early twenties, I began teaching in an after-school program in a settlement house in Chicago's inner city. I made up learning games to make reading, writing, science and other subjects fun. When I began teaching yoga, I found that I was much better at it when I was teaching it. By sharing it with others, I took my mind off myself and my body relaxed and became suppler. I was filled with a special glow and energy after our yoga classes.

Later, I was hired to start a children's yoga program at the Chicago Yoga Institute, where I took courses and was certified. I wonder how many people my first teacher reached through her magical television show? I wonder how many people her students have reached? How many people will you reach in your teaching practice?

—Matthew Calhoun
Astoria, New York

I. Introduction

What allows kids to use a lot of energy, make funny noises, relax, and learn to focus all at the same time? It is yoga. For kids to gain the full benefits of yoga, there needs to be a flow and an overall plan to the practice. *Create a Yoga Practice for Kids: Fun, Flexibility, and Focus* is a book designed to give everyone confidence in yoga practice and to increase the kids' involvement.

Creating a 45 minute practice is as easy as 1-2-3 by choosing one group of poses from three sections:

1) Opening Poses stretch and awaken the muscles with movement and breath, while bringing the focus to yoga.

2) Themes provide a sequence of interactive, energizing poses.

3) Relaxation Poses offer a calming way to end the practice.

Waterfall Pose

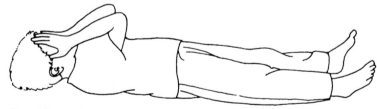

Eye Warming

The "More Yoga Fun" section provides a variety of extension activities including a five-minute yoga break for the classroom, yoga games, more visualization exercises, and yoga to do at a wall. These are not necessary to complete the 45-minute practice but are offered as options to keep your practices lively.

The Chain Game

What is Yoga?

Yoga is an art and a science. The word yoga is from the Sanskrit word *yuj,* which means the yoking or joining of two things, "whatever their nature".(1) It can be joining the body with the mind or joining of the individual with some larger entity. As A.G. Mohan explains in his book, *Yoga for Body, Breath, and Mind*, the joining represents a process. Practicing yoga is not just completing a pose because yoga also includes what happens along the way. It includes such things as how you breathe, how you are listening to your body, and how your mind is focused on what you are doing now, in the present. Yoga poses, or *asanas*, work to strengthen the body and to calm the mind by using the breath.

Yoga was developed in India thousands of years ago and was committed to writing by Pantajali in the *Yoga Sutras* over 2,000 years ago. Yoga integrates physical movement and spiritual growth. Yoga is not a specific religion or set of beliefs. The Yoga Sutras define yoga as "the process of channeling the activities of the mind in the desired direction, and sustaining that focus without being distracted."

Like science, one comes to know yoga through what one experiences. And from one's yoga practice comes personal growth and awareness—at any age.

How does yoga benefit kids?

Kids can derive many of the same benefits from yoga that adults do. Yoga heals and strengthens a person in many ways. Part of yoga is physical exercise. In fact, it is an activity included in the President's Challenge Program, part of the President's Council on Physical Fitness and Sports. Yoga helps build muscles, coordination, flexibility, and stamina. Like other exercise, yoga provides a physical release for stress.

But yoga offers more than just physical exercise. As young people practice yoga, they can increase their self-confidence and their ability to concentrate and to focus. Yoga also fosters creativity and self-expression as children explore and develop their own variations on poses.

Practicing yoga teaches kids how to relax and how to deal with stress by using breathing techniques and imagery strategies. Learning how to relax is a key to physical and mental health.

The use of breathing techniques to lower stress levels and blood pressure is becoming more commonly used in part because of the important work of such doctors as Dean Ornish and Herbert Benson.(2)(3) A few simple breath exercises for children can teach them to use their breath, something they can always find, to calm themselves. As Donna Farhi says, "Becoming attuned to your breath is like learning to dance the waltz with a partner."(4)

Nischala Joy Devi explains in *The Healing Path of Yoga* that imagery can be used to actively create a situation or form an idea in one's mind.(5) One can imagine different senses (seeing, hearing, tasting, feeling) to develop images in the mind. Guiding children through simple visualization exercises introduces them to ways they can find their own state of relaxation.

Who can do yoga?

"Yoga is for everyone," says Yogacharya B.K.S. Iyengar, one of the world's leading yoga teachers.(6) This does not mean that every person can or should do every pose. It means that there are some yoga poses that everyone can enjoy, whatever your level of fitness or age.

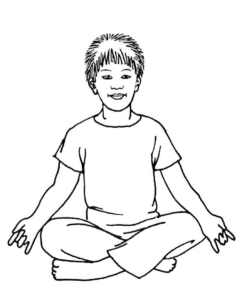

The poses in this book are designed for those new to yoga, but more advanced poses also are offered. The benefits of yoga—relaxation, muscle strengthening and flexibility, focus, and self-confidence—are also beneficial for many special needs children.

Caution: If someone is known to have a specific medical condition, a doctor should be consulted before involving that person in any type of yoga practice.

Easy Pose

What do I need to practice yoga?

Many yoga poses can be done on a floor, a carpet, or even outdoors with no props or equipment. It is more comfortable to have a yoga mat or a large towel on an uncarpeted floor for the poses done lying down. Listening to gentle music creates a relaxing atmosphere, but it is not necessary. Soft music in the background allows the teacher to gain everyone's attention by simply saying, "Listen for the music." A brief pause with the hands in prayer pose to listen for the music never fails to refocus the attention!

Why is a sequence of poses important to a practice?

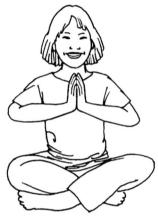

Creating a practice with a definite beginning, middle, and end makes many of the benefits of yoga available to kids. Sequencing of poses allows you to warm up the muscles groups and to set a tone for the practice. Opening warm-up poses are followed by the more dynamic, active poses that create the theme for the practice. A theme keeps the kids involved as they try to guess what is coming next. Sequencing also allows you to work certain muscles groups and then to do a counterpose that releases the muscles. Finally, there should be a time in the practice for the body and mind to grow calm. Ending with a relaxation section allows people to explore the restorative aspect of yoga.

Easy Pose

Since sequencing the poses is important, is it helpful to write out the practice?

We would encourage you to find what works for you. When Yael first started teaching, she had a clipboard in front of her mat with the sequence written in dark marker so she could easily see it. After she became familiar with the sequences, she stopped doing that. She noticed a change in the class! They thought she didn't have a plan, and the kids started trying to run the class themselves, always interrupting with what they wanted to do next. While Yael appreciated their enthusiasm, she brought back the clipboard prop, explaining that there would be a time at the end of the class for doing their favorites or the poses they developed. Without stifling their excitement or creativity, she still maintained the flow. You may want to write one or two ideas from the following "Suggestion for What to Say" section on the paper just as a reminder. Add a new one each practice.

Matthew prefers to work with nothing written out, committing to memory what he is going to do and varying it spontaneously as he listens to his body and the class. Different styles work for different teachers.

How long do we hold a pose?

The focus in yoga is on the breath, not on minutes ticking by, so poses are held for a number of breaths. For children, two or three series of inhales and exhales is beneficial.

How do I keep the kids' attention?

There are some tried and true ways to hold kids' interest. One way is to ask them questions, many of which are offered in the "Suggestions for What to Say" section. In Butterfly Pose, ask them where they are flying. In Cat Pose, ask why the cat is angry and hissing. In Tree Pose, ask what kind of tree they are. You can quickly draw a person into the practice by showing that you know his name and care what he is thinking.

Another way to keep attention during the theme section is to ask how the next pose might look—how would Down Dog look if we turned it upside down (Boat Pose)? How would Chair Pose look if we doubled it?

After you have demonstrated the pose, perhaps using a person as a model in the front of the room, move about and help people. Make positive comments. "Your body really likes yoga," or "You make that look like your favorite pose," are examples. It is not helpful to say, "That looks great!" since you may easily make someone else feel that they do not look great. Yoga is about how it FEELS, not how it looks.

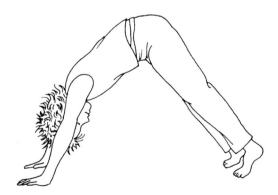

Down Dog

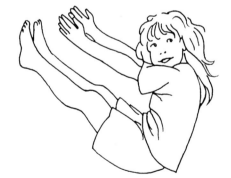

Boat Pose

Do I need to use the *Sanskrit* names?

Using the *Sanskrit* name for a pose is not necessary. However, using some *Sanskrit* names can add a nice flavor to the practice. Kids love the sounds of words, and *Sanskrit* names have wonderful sounds. In addition, it gives everyone a sense of being in a special club that uses a special language to show membership. We have included some *Sanskrit* names, and a pronunciation guide is found in Appendix A.

What is helpful to say during the practice?

Teaching yoga to kids is much different than teaching yoga to adults, although the benefits are similar. Kids do not want to listen to you talking *at* them about how to do the poses and the benefits of yoga. Kids like to move around and to make silly noises.

It is important to find a balance—give the kids a general idea of the pose, let them try it, and then give them a pointer or two. A fun yoga practice has to be interactive, meaning you must interact with the kids and allow them space to interact with you. You can keep the structure of the practice and still be open to their ideas. It is appropriate to say, "Let's try that at the end when we do our favorites," or "That's a fun idea, let's try that right after we finish this pose."

To ensure that the kids get the benefits of yoga, the practice needs to maintain its yoga focus. Otherwise, it becomes an exercise class, which has benefits—but not those of yoga. You can easily teach a yoga practice and still have a lot of fun.

Begin standing in the front of the room to introduce a pose. It can be helpful to have a child volunteer in the front with you to help you demonstrate. Then you are free to move around the room and help others.

Here are some ideas about what to say throughout a practice.

1. Move with your breath.

"Yoga is about moving with your breath. We breathe in and then start to move. The breath gives us a focus point. When our mind gets too busy with other thoughts, we can just watch our breath. Do not change it—just watch and observe it. Breath connects the body to the mind and helps to calm us. That is why we tell people who are upset to take a deep breath. In yoga, we breathe in through the nose."

Note: With every pose, mention the breath. Before you start a pose, have everyone take a deep inhale, and as they move into the pose, everyone should slowly release the breath, or exhale. When you release from a pose, do it in a flowing style, like the breath. In yoga, breath is inhaled through the nose. It warms, slows, and cleans the breath.**(7)**

2.   Listen to your body.

"This yoga practice is for you. Only you can listen to your body from inside yourself. When you need to rest, go into Child's Pose. When you are ready to join us again, your body will let you know. Taking a little break will help you to enjoy the rest of the practice."

"If it hurts, don't do it. It is good to feel a little stretch in the muscles, but it is not good to feel any pain. We move slowly in and out of the poses, so we can listen to what our bodies are telling us."

Note: Presenting the idea in this way helps the kids to develop a sense of control over their bodies in different situations. Such control is a key to managing stress and learning to relax.

3.   Listen for the music

"Let's listen for the music. Stand with your hands folded, your thumbs pressing into your chest. Lightly press your palms together in prayer pose. Close your eyes and listen for the music. Take several breaths here."

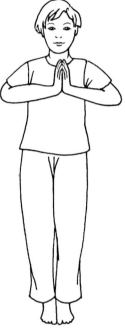

Listen for the Music

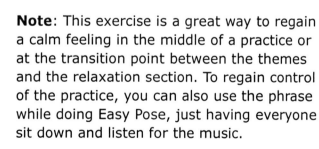

Note: This exercise is a great way to regain a calm feeling in the middle of a practice or at the transition point between the themes and the relaxation section. To regain control of the practice, you can also use the phrase while doing Easy Pose, just having everyone sit down and listen for the music.

Listen for the Music

4.   You are doing yoga only for yourself.

"Yoga is a gift you are giving to yourself. You are not doing it to impress anyone, so do not compare yourself to someone else. What matters is what *you* are doing and what *you* are feeling, not how you look or how the person next to you looks."

5.   Yoga feels good.

"Sometimes moving slowly in and out of a pose feels good. It creates a flowing and dynamic feeling. The second time you do a pose is usually easier as the muscles warm and stretch. And one side may be easier to do than the other."

6.   Be positive!

"Some poses may not work for you. You can tell yourself that maybe today you are not going to do this pose. But while we do it, in your mind *imagine* yourself doing it. A first step is imagining it or having the intention of doing the pose. Tell yourself that sometime, maybe next week or next month, you may do this pose. Just not right now. And that is okay."

Note: If there is a pose you did not learn easily, you could share this as an example. Perhaps it took you a while before you could do Crow—kids like to know that adults practice too.

7.   This pose is very good for...

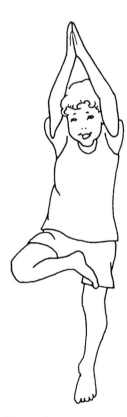

"Practicing Tree Pose helps us to build focus and concentration. Balance poses like Tree Pose are great to do before you study or practice an instrument. It clears your mind—the only thing you can be thinking about is not falling!"

Note: Benefits are explained after each pose description. Only mention one benefit for each pose, or your comments can be distracting. As poses have more than one benefit, you can mention a different one each time. Kids will get the message that yoga does a lot of different things for them. We have offered a muscle or muscle group that a pose work—mentioning it gives the kids a sense of their bodies' involvement.
"Let me know when you feel your leg (or arm) muscles working in this pose!"

Tree Pose

8.   What else could we do?

A wonderful way to keep the practice interactive is to ask people to think of another pose for next week that might fit in with the theme we are doing today. Or you can encourage them to develop their own poses (like Wolf Pose, which was developed by a Fifth grader) to share at the end of a practice.

Kids also come up with wonderful new theme ideas as they become more familiar with the poses. Someone came up with a "Favorites Day" theme, in which everyone gets to choose their favorite pose for us to do. Yoga is about exploring, so use the opportunity to explore yoga with your kids.

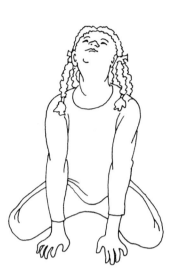

Wolf Pose

A Final Note

Remember, yoga is a wonderful gift you are giving to kids. It is a tool they can keep with them always. Perhaps they won't become yogis, but at a future time they may remember that yoga provided them with something they need: a way to have fun and a way to find some peace.

> *In everyone's life, at some time, our inner*
> *fire goes out. It is then burst into flame*
> *by an encounter with another human*
> *being. We should all be thankful for those*
> *people who rekindle the inner spirit.*
> —Albert Schweitzer (1875–1965)

Namaste.

II. Opening Poses

Amusing poses are a great way to begin a practice. Making kids smile or laugh immediately draws their focus to what you are doing. Opening poses also begin to warm and stretch the muscles, which is important before engaging in more energizing poses.

Suggestions for What to Say:

A.　　Sequence 1

1.　　Color-the-Room

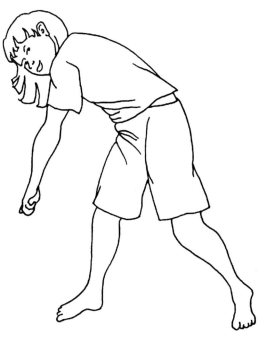

"Yoga is a wonderful way to stretch your mind and body. Let's play a yoga game called Color-the-Room. Reach out your hand and pretend to grab your favorite color crayon. As you breathe in, stretch your hand over your head as high as you can and draw three big, colorful circles. Feel the stretch on your sides. What colors do you see on the ceiling? Now draw in the opposite direction. Put that arm down, and raise the other arm and grab a color that makes you feel silly. Again, stretch up high and make three wide circles in each direction. How does the ceiling look?"

Color-the-Room

"Now, let's do the walls. Reach a hand out and grab a color that makes you feel happy. What color makes you feel happy? Draw a big circle reaching from over your head to the floor. As you move up, breathe in through your nose. As you move down, breathe out and bend your knees so they are soft. Do this three times, and then we can change colors and reverse direction."

"Then with the other hand, reach out and grab a color that makes you feel quiet. Draw the three circles, remembering to breathe. Now how does the room look?"

Benefits: Opening with something silly allows the kids to feel the fun in yoga. It is a nice way to bring everyone together before formally beginning the practice with Easy Pose.

2.   Easy Pose (*Sukhasana*)

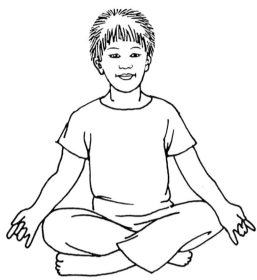

Easy Pose

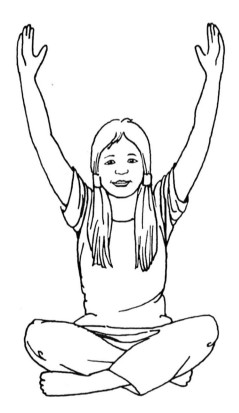

Breathing Exercise in Easy Pose

"Sit in Easy Pose by folding your legs in front of you. Sit with a tall spine and roll your shoulders back. Gently rock to each side and find your comfortable seat."

Benefits: Sitting with a tall spine is relaxing and makes it easier to breathe. Easy Pose is a good pose to do again in the middle of a practice, just to bring the focus back to the breath and to a state of calm as they absorb the benefits of yoga.

a.   Set Intentions:

"Now close your eyes and set your intention for the class: it could be that you want to relax, to stretch, to spend time with a friend, do something nice for yourself, or to learn something new. When your intention is set, open your eyes."

Note: You may want to offer an intention that considers a yoga idea. *Santosha* is a *Sanksrit* word that means contentment. The intention for this practice could be for you to find contentment in the way you are doing a pose. Sometimes when we are always striving to do better we lose sight of the pleasure of where we are now. While it is good to have goals, we can lose a lot if we do not attend to where we are now.

Benefits: Setting an intention before you start a practice lets the kids know that they have some control over what yoga does for them.

b.   Breathing (*Pranayama*) Exercise

"An important part of yoga is the breath. We keep an awareness of our breathing and move with the breath. As you take a deep breath in through the nose, raise your arms over your head. Breathe in the good energy from those around you who have come to do yoga with you. As you lower your hands, breathe out anything that is bothering you, any tense feelings or troubled thoughts, any little aches and pains."

Note: Repeat this three times.

Benefits: The kids love this part—I hear murmurs of, "Oh yeah, my math test," and similar comments. It gives them a chance to "step away" from their days.

c.   Seated Twist

"Now we're going to take a break and by doing some seated twists. Place your right hand on the outside of your left knee. Reach your left hand out in front of you, take a deep breath in through your nose. As you breathe out, gently clear the space with your hand as turn to look over your left shoulder. Take another breath in, and as you breathe out, move into the twist a little bit more, even a centimeter. Then slowly come back to center. Yoga is also about balance, so what we do on one side, we then do on the other. Let's repeat this gentle twist on the other side."

Note: You may want to repeat this, asking the students if they feel they can twist a little more the second time.

Benefits: Twists provide a gentle squeezing of the internal organs, like the kidneys, intestines, and liver. When you come out of the twist, the organs are infused with fresh blood and cleansed.

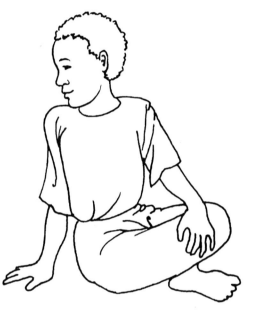

Seated Twist

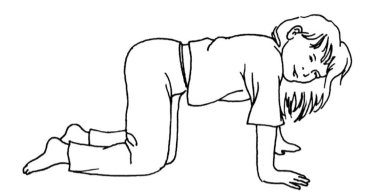

Flatback

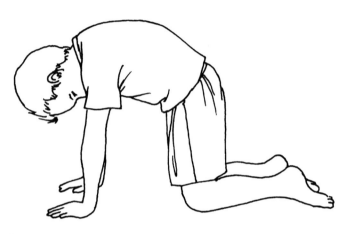

Cat Pose

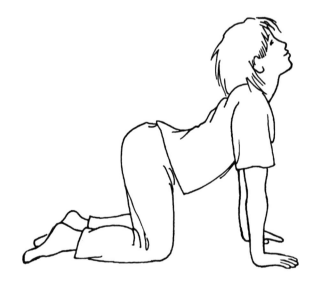

Cow pose

3. Cat/Cow/Puppy Wag Sequence

a. Cat/Cow

"Animals have a lot of wisdom in their bodies, and you do, too. We need to get our spines warmed up before we start doing other poses. Get on your hands and knees with your hands under your shoulders and your knees under your hips (flatback). Take a deep breath, and as you breathe out, arch your back and drop your head and hiss like a fierce cat. Why is the cat feeling fierce?

Take another breath and lift your back a little higher. Breathe out and come back to Flatback. Take a breath in through your nose as you drop your back and raise your head like an old cow. Give a sorry-sounding "moooo" as you drop your back a little more. Why is the cow feeling so sad and sorry?"

Note: Repeat this three times. It is very fun to do this facing one or two people.

Benefits: It is important to keep your spine flexible. Doing the cat/cow sequence wakes up your spine by providing an easy bend in both directions.

b. Puppy Wag

"Find your Flatback Pose again. Let's stretch our spines in the other direction. Pretend you have a puppy dog tail that is wagging. Without moving your hips, take a deep breath in, and as you push the breath out, look over your left shoulder at your wiggling puppy tail. Give puppy yips as you go. Let's do this on the other side."

Note: Repeat one or two more times.

Benefits: This pose provides a lateral stretch to the spine. It is not the way we usually stretch, and it provides a good balance to the cat/cow spinal stretch.

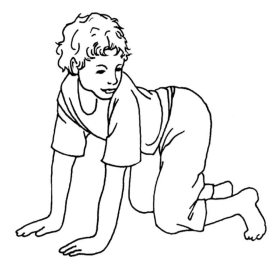

Puppy Wag

c. Pick-a-Pose

"Now pick any of these three poses that you really like and do it again, making the right animal sound as you do. Then we will all meet in a quiet Flatback. Now choose the pose that did not work that well for you, and try it again. See if it works better for your body this time."

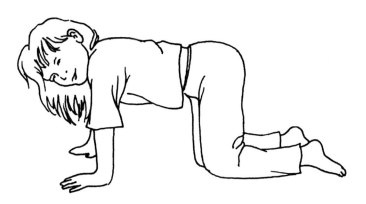

Flatback

Benefits: A person's body is different every day. Certain poses may feel good one day, and not another. Doing the Pick-a-Pose exercise introduces children to the idea that you can explore a pose (or anything else) and perhaps find things to like about it.

4.   Flatback Balance Pose (Nose-to-Knee)

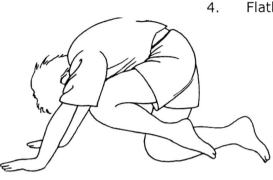

Flatback Nose-to-Knee

"Practicing balance helps you to become better balanced and build concentration. Before you study for a test or if you are trying to focus on something, it helps to do some balance poses first. Find Flatback Pose again. As you breathe in through your nose, reach your right hand out in front of you. Lift your left leg and press back as though there were a wall in back of you. You can stay here for several breaths"

"Stay in this pose if it feels good. But you may want to push all your breath out as pull your left leg in and bend your head down so that your left knee touches your nose!"

Note: Do the knee-to-nose two times as you breathe in and out with the each movement. Then do the other side.

Benefits: This pose builds balance and develops concentration. It also gives kids a sense that yoga has a flow.

5.   Child's Pose *(Balasana)*

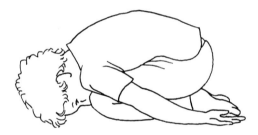

Child's Pose

"Did you know that your body can be absorbing and learning things while you rest? Find Flatback Pose and then sit back on your heels. Rest your arms down by your side or out in front of you. You can come into this pose to rest at any time during the practice. Then, when your body is ready, you can join us in what we are doing. Yoga teaches us that it is important to listen to our bodies."

Note: You can practice Child's Pose with your arms by your feet or with your arms stretched to the front. Try it both ways and notice how it relaxes or stretches different muscles.

Benefits: Child's Pose is a resting pose that provides a gentle backstretch, while releasing the muscles in the lower back. It is important for kids to know they can rest when they need to. Some poses are tiring and a two-minute break, when they decide, prevents the kids from losing interest or giving up when a pose does not serve them.

B. Sequence 2

1. Lion Pose

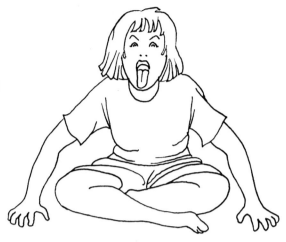

"Doing this silly pose can help you fight off a sore throat or just give you some energy. Do you know how far away a lion cub can hear his mama lion roar? Five miles!"

"Sit back on your heels with your toes tucked under. Open your mouth as wide as you can, stick out your tongue as far as you can, and roar as loud as you can. Now watch me."

"I am not sure the lion cub could hear you. Let's try that again."

Lion Pose

Benefits: Lion Pose stimulates the lymph regions in the head and neck. It is also a great way to get everyone's attention focused on yoga because it is a funny, noisy pose to do.

2. Easy Pose (*Sukhasana*)

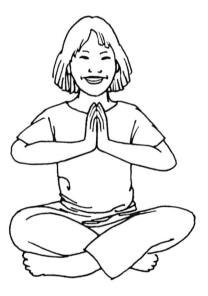

"Here is a fun way to stretch your spine—you may even leave here a little taller today. Let's sit with our legs folded comfortably. Roll your shoulders back and sit up tall. Let your body move until you feel 'easy'. Fold your hands into Prayer Pose and gently press your thumbs into your chest. Now close your eyes."

Benefits: Easy Pose shows the kids that yoga has a calming side. It serves as a balance to the funny opening pose.

Easy Pose

a.   Set Intentions:

"Let's set an intention for our practice. It could be that you want to relax, to stretch, to spend time with a friend, do something nice for yourself, or to learn something new. When your intention is set, open your eyes."

Note: Another idea to think about in setting an intention is that of *mudita*—finding happiness in the joy or good fortune of others. Instead of getting angry or jealous, practicing *mudita* can help an individual develop a positive mindset and stop losing energy to negative feelings.

Benefits: Setting an intention gives people a chance to consider that their yoga practice has a purpose.

b.   Bellows Breathing (*pranayama*) exercise:

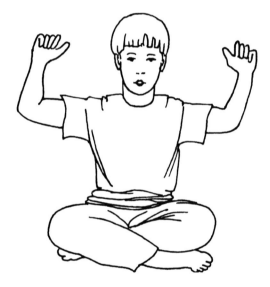

"How much air can you blow out of your lungs? Take a deep breath as you raise your arms up high, then blow all the air out of your lungs as you drop your arms down to your side! Can you blow a little more air out through your nose? Imagine you are blowing out any thoughts, feeling, or distractions that are bothering you."

Benefits: Developing an awareness of the breath is a key to the calming effect of yoga. This exercise is a fun way to begin that awareness.

c.   Head/Shoulder/Wrist Rolls

Bellows Breathing

"Imagine you have a brightly colored pencil on the tip of your nose. Use that pencil to slowly draw an infinity sign or the number eight lying on its side. We are going to do this three times in one direction. Then come back to center and change the color of your pencil. Gently draw the figure going in the other direction. Do it three times."

"Now lift your shoulders up toward your ears. Roll them back and down, and back up again in the front—three times toward the back and then three times toward the front."

"Hold your arms out over your knees. Pretend each finger can draw a different color. Without moving your arms, roll your wrists around so your fingers draw big circles. Do this three times in each direction

Benefits: Gentle movement of the head relaxes the neck muscles. A human head weighs over five pounds, which is a lot for neck muscles to hold up. Shoulder and wrist rolls help to lubricate the joints in these areas.

3.   Butterfly Pose *(Baddha Konasana)*

"Close your eyes and imagine a special place you would like to fly. Take a deep breath and imagine the smells. Take another breath and imagine the sounds."

"Sit with your spine straight. Roll your shoulders back so your chest is ready to receive a deep breath. Pull your legs in so that the soles of your feet touch. If this hurts your knees, keep the soles of your feet together, but move them down the mat. Remember, a pose should never cause you pain. Now take a deep inhale through your nose, and as you release your breath, raise your knees about six inches off the floor. Gently raise and lower your knees, just as though your legs were butterfly wings. Close your eyes again and imagine you are flying to your special spot. I would like to fly to see flowering cactus in the spring. Where would you like to fly as a butterfly?

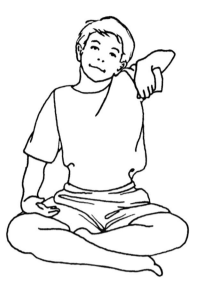

Head/Shoulder/Wrist Rolls

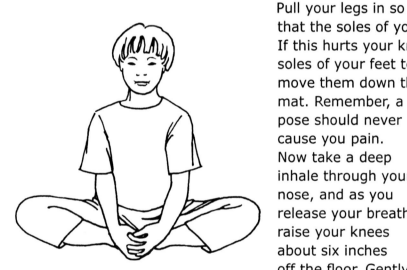

Butterfly Pose

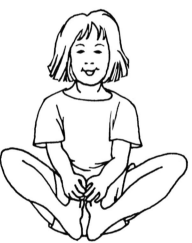

Butterfly Pose

Benefits: This pose opens the muscles in the inner thighs and the hips. It also helps to keep the knees, feet, and ankles flexible. It also helps kids to practice visualization.

4.   Rock-the-Baby

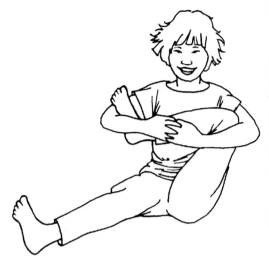
Rock-the-Baby

"How many of you have ever held a baby? Babies love to be rocked. Let's see how it feels to pretend your leg is a baby you can rock."

"Sit in Easy Pose. Now, hold your right foot with your left hand. Put your right hand on your right knee. Slowly raise your right foot so that it sits in the crook of your left elbow. Bring your hands together under your leg, as if you are rocking a baby. Stay focused on your right leg, as you gently move your arms back and forth. What does that leg feel like, as it is cradled and protected? Gently release your leg to the floor. Let's do the other side. This time as you rock your leg, pay attention to how you can breathe in and out through your nose as you rock."

Note: You can also try this from a lying down position.

Benefits: This pose is a good warm-up pose because it gently stretches the hip.

5.   Downward Facing Dog (Down Dog) to Childs' Pose to Cobra

a.   Downward Facing Dog (*Adho Mukha Svanasana*)

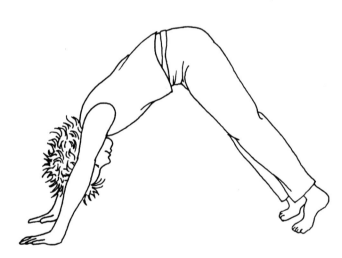
Down Dog

"We are going to finish our warm-up with a flow of three poses. How many of you ever watched a dog? Maybe you have seen her do this pose—it's called 'Down Dog'. It's a good wake-up pose because a lot of muscles get stretched and your brain gets a lot of fresh blood. Get on your hands and knees with a flat back. Your hands are right under your shoulders. Curl your toes under and push your hips up. Feel as though someone has a belt around your hips and is pulling you toward the sky. Stretch your heels down toward the mat. Let's stay here while we take a deep breath in through our nose and then push the breath out. Now lower your knees to the floor and sit back on your heels."

36

Benefits: Down Dog is a great shoulder stretch. It helps lengthen your spine and stretch the hamstring and calf muscles in the backs of your legs. In addition, it also allows extra blood to go to the head, bringing oxygen and nutrients to the brain.

b.   Child's Pose (*Balasana*)

"You probably did this pose when you slept as a baby. Let's see if it still makes you feel peaceful. It is a pose you can do anytime during a practice when you choose to take a little break."

"Sit back on your heels and rest your head on the floor. Find a place that feels restful for your arms. Let any concerns you have just roll off your back. Think of your back as a hard turtle shell protecting you. Take a deep breath and settle into your comfortable place."

"If you are ever feeling upset or nervous, you can picture in your mind that you are doing this pose. Sometimes just imagining yourself doing a yoga pose can make you feel better."

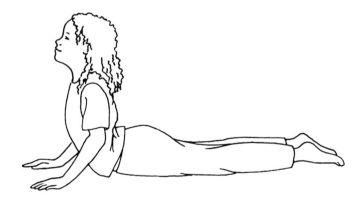

Benefits: This pose shows kids that they can give comfort and rest to themselves. It also shows that a pause in a practice is a good habit.

Child's Pose

c.   Cobra

"Now scoop your head through, letting your chin touch the mat as you flatten out your body and gently raise your head, like a spitting cobra. As you come through the pose, hiss like a snake. Do snakes have arms? Can you lift your arms off the mat and still hold yourself up. Squeeze the muscles in your seat together to support your lower back. The next time you breathe out, push yourself back into Down Dog so that we can do the series one more time."

Benefits: Cobra strengthens the lower back. It also opens the chest so you can breathe more deeply.

Cobra

C. Sequence 3

1. Mountain Pose (*Tadasana*)
a. Stretch Up

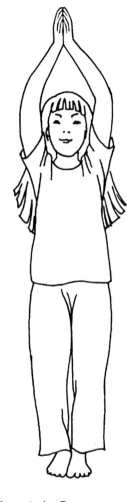

Mountain Pose

"We are going to stand like a tall mountain. Find a comfortable place for your feet and gently rock back and forth to find the point where you feel balanced and strong, like the rocky base of a mountain. Roll your shoulders back, keep your eyes looking forward. Take a deep breath in through your nose as your hands up and reach for the clouds."

"Look up at your hands and imagine they are snow covered mountain peaks. What is a high mountain you know? Now imagine the sun melting the snow. As the snow melts and the streams run down your body, anything that is bothering you is washed away in the clear, cool, mountain water."

b. Set Intentions

"Now lower your hands into Prayer Pose. Spread your fingers and feel your thumbs press into your chest as you close your eyes. Now we can set an intention for the class: it could be that you want to relax, to learn how to concentrate better, to spend time with a friend, do something nice for yourself, or to learn something new. When you have set your intention, open your eyes."

Note: Another idea for a personal intention is to think about the yoga idea of *ahimsa*, or non-harming. Not harming, or not hurting, has to start with oneself. So people can think about being nice to themselves during this practice, and then take that idea with them when they leave.

Benefits: Setting an intention brings attention to the fact that yoga practice is about to begin—and there is a plan.

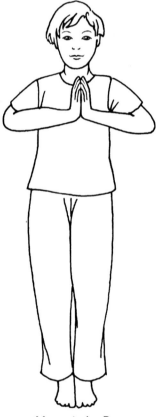

*Mountain Pose:
Hands in Prayer*

c.   Moving With the Breath

"An important part of yoga is moving with your breath. That's one reason that just jumping around at recess is not yoga. Yoga does so many good things for your body and your mind, so let's begin our yoga practice by moving with the breath. As you inhale, or breathe in through your nose, let your arms flow up over your head. When you exhale, or breathe out, let your arms melt back to your sides. Think about your breath as a wave, and your movement is riding the wave. Let's do this three times. You can follow me, or you can move with your own breath."

Benefits: Moving with the breath, or aligning the breath with our movement, is what yoga is all about. Doing this pose with a conscious connection to the breath allows kids to explore what "moving with the breath" means.

2.   Tree Pose (*Vrksasana*)

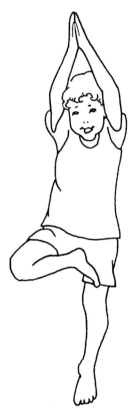

Tree Pose

"Who has a favorite tree? Does it keep its leaves all year like an evergreen, or do the leaves change colors in the fall? There are many different kinds of trees, and there are many different ways to do this pose."
    First, look straight across the room and find something at eye level that is not moving. You can focus on this spot, which is called a *drishti* point."
    "Now stand in Mountain Pose. Imagine roots growing down into the earth to anchor your left foot. Lift your right foot as much as you like: you can place your toes on the floor next to your leg, you can lean your right foot against your left calf, or even tuck your right foot into your left thigh. If you do this, press your thigh into your foot – both legs are active and pressing firmly against each other so you have a solid base. Now breathe your arms up and reach for the sky, like a giant sequoia. Gently wave your arms, like a maple blowing in the wind. Now let your arms droop down like a weeping willow. Let your right leg come down to meet your left. Find your mountain again, and then grow a tree on the other side."
Note: Kids can lean a hand on a friend's shoulder or use the wall to practice. You can even make a forest of trees. After the kids are familiar with Tree Pose, add the wonderful Tree Poem game found on page 119.

Benefits: Tree pose helps to build balance and develop focus. It also is a great stretch for the whole body.

3.   Flatback/Arm Balance Flow

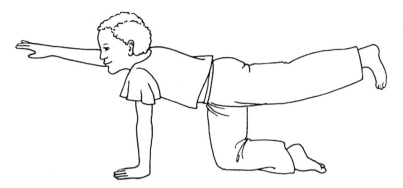

"Did you know that you are all great at balancing on very small things? You balance all day long on your feet! Let's see how well we can balance with more of our bodies on the floor. Let's include a hand in the balance too."

"Begin on your hands and knees. Take a

Flatback/Arm Balance

deep breath in and reach your right hand out in front of you. As we breathe out, let's raise our left leg and stretch it back. Bring your hand and leg down, and let's try balancing on the other side."

Note: A challenge is to balance with the right hand and right leg both extended.

Benefits: This pose is energizing and starts to build some heat in the body so the muscles can stretch and lengthen more easily. It also helps to develop balance and concentration.

4.   Child's Pose (*Balasana*)

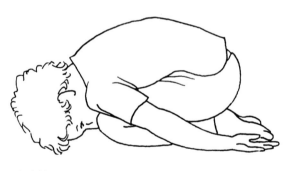

"All babies need a lot of rest because they are growing so quickly and need to save their energy for growing new cells. Let's give our bodies a rest as we are growing too."

"Find Flatback Pose and then sit back on your heels. Rest your arms down by your side or out in front of you. Please find Child's Pose anytime you need to gather your energy."

Child's Pose

Benefits: Child's Pose allows the kids to take a break from external stimulation and absorb the benefits of a pause in the day.

III.   Themes

Having a theme to your day's practice keeps everyone's attention. They try to guess what the opposite pose is, and as they get more familiar with the yoga poses, they will add their own creative suggestions. Kids have a natural sense of yoga, and they enjoy creating new sequences and poses.

Suggestions for What to Say:

A.   Theme 1: Opposites

Thinking about things in a different way can give us new ideas. Looking at the world from upside down can give us a new perspective too. It is good to give kids an opportunity to experience things from a new angle!

1.   Plank Pose to Slide Pose

a.   Plank Pose

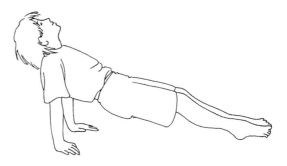

Plank Pose

"Let's make our bodies look like planks, or boards that are so straight we could draw a line from your head, across your spine, and down your legs."
    "Start on your hands and knees. Curl your toes under, slowly straighten your legs, and lift your hips. Take a deep breath and see if you can feel your breath move in that straight line down to your toes."

b.   Slide Pose

"Picture in your mind how the opposite of Plank Pose would look.
    Come down to your knees, and then sit back on your feet. Straighten your legs out in front of you. Lean back on your arms with your fingers pointing toward your seat. On your next breath in through your nose, push up and raise your hips off the mat. Can you take another deep breath and move your breath along the straight line from your head, across your stomach, down to your toes?"
    "Slowly lower yourself down to the earth."

Slide Pose

Benefits: These poses build strength in the arms, shoulders, and wrists. They also help to lengthen the spine.

2. Downward Facing Dog to Boat Pose
a. Downward Facing Dog (*Adho Mukha Svanasana*)

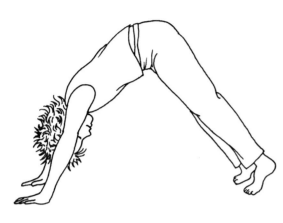

Down Dog

"How many of you know a dog? You may have seen the dog do this pose after she gets up from a nap. That's why it is called Down Dog."

"Let's start on our hands and knees with a flat back. Your paws are right under your shoulders. Curl your toes under, push your hips up, and reach your bottom up to the sky. Stretch your heels down toward the mat. What shape are we making? Let's stay here for several breaths. Now lower your knees to the floor and sit back on your heels and rest."

Benefits: Down Dog is a great shoulder stretch. It also helps you to lengthen your spine and stretch the hamstring and calf muscles in the backs of your legs. In addition, it also allows extra blood to go to the head, bringing oxygen and nutrients to the brain

b. Boat Pose (*Navasana*)

"How could we make the 'V' shape of Down Dog go in the opposite way? What is sticking up in the air when we are in Down Dog? That is the part of our body we need to have on the floor now."

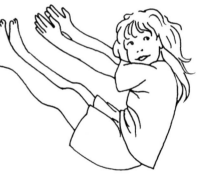

Boat Pose

"Sit with your legs out in front of you. Bend your knees and lift your legs off the mat. You can wrap your arms around your legs if that helps you to find a balance spot on your seat! Can you stretch your arms out in front of you? If it feels good, you can straighten your legs so your body is in a "V" shape. Remember, you can bend your knees if that feels better—listen to your body."

Benefits: Boat Pose builds strength in the abdominal muscles. It is also a great pose for practicing balance, which in turn builds concentration!

3.   Snowball Pose to Star Pose
a.   Snowball Pose

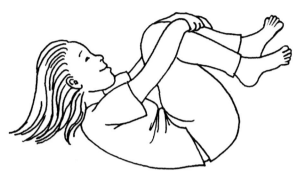

"Snowball is a silly pose because we roll our bodies around like snowballs."

"Lie on your back, pull your knees into your chest, and wrap your arms around your legs. Pull your head up so your body is in a tight ball. Now you can either rock from side to side, or you can rock with more energy so that your body moves around in a circle. We are going to do this three times in each direction. See how big you can make your snowball!"

Snowball Pose

Benefits: Snowball Pose gently releases the muscles in the lower back and massages the internal organs. It also makes everyone laughs, which lowers stress hormone levels.

b.   Star Pose

"We were just rolling around in a tight ball. How could we do the opposite with our bodies?"

"Let's stand up and spread our feet apart. Press your feet into the earth. Let's raise our arms and reach out, as if someone is gently pulling our arms into space. Raise your head tall. Now everything is spreading your energy out, like a star burning bright and hot. Take a deep inhale through the nose and slowly release the breath."

Note: Repeat twice.

Benefits: This pose energizes the body and provides a good stretch for the legs, shoulders, and arms. It also opens the chest, which allows for deeper breathing.

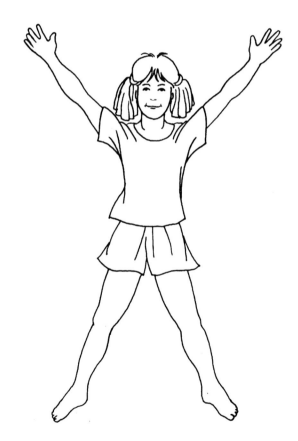

Star Pose

4. Warrior 2 to Reverse Warrior 2
a. Warrior 2 (*Virabhadrasana* 2)

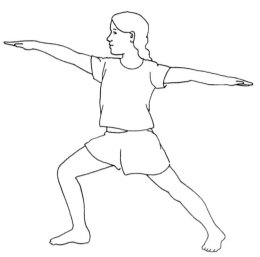

Warrior 2

"Warrior poses are not done to hurt anyone, they are done to make you feel strong and powerful."

"Stand with your legs apart, about the distance of one of your legs. Turn your toes in slightly, like a duck. Since you are standing like a duck, maybe you can quack three times like a duck too! Now turn your right foot so that it points forward. As you take a deep inhale, breathe your arms up. Your two arms now look like one straight arm. Look out over your right hand. Now see if you can bend your right leg—only go down as far as feels good."

Note: Make sure the right knee does not extend over the right foot, which can damage the knee. The left hip comes forward a little in this pose.

Benefits: This pose energizes the body and provides a good stretch for the legs, shoulders, and arms. It also opens the chest, which allows for deeper breathing.

b. Reverse Warrior 2

"We can put this pose in reverse by moving our arms. Slide your left arm down toward your back leg. Breathe in and as you breathe, sweep your right arm over your head in a gentle arc. Let's take another breath and move back to Warrior 2. Now on your next exhale, or breath out, sweep your arms back in Reverse Warrior 2."

Note: Repeat this three times.

Benefits: Reverse Warrior 2 is an energizing pose. It strengthens the legs and provides a good stretch to the side of the body.

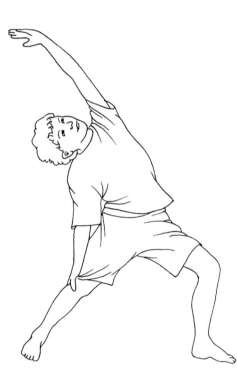

Reverse Warrior 2

5.   Bow Pose to Bridge Pose

a.   Bow Pose *(Dhanurasana)*

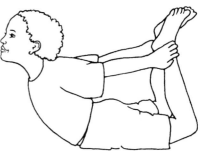

"How do you think it feels to stretch and be strong at the same time? Let's find out as we stretch out like a bow that is about to shoot an arrow."

"Lie on your stomach and stretch out your hands and legs. Raise your right foot and reach around and grab the top of your right foot with your right hand. Now raise your left foot and grab it with your left hand. Your body is the wooden part of the bow, being stretched tight before the arrow is released. Your arms are the bowstring."

Bow Pose

"As you breathe out, kick your feet into your hands as you lift your arms. Remember, if this hurts your knees, come down! As you exhale again, release down to the floor and relax for two breaths. Let's do this again."

Benefits: This is an energizing pose. It stretches the abdominal muscles and strengthens all the muscles in the back. It is a good pose to do after sitting all day.

b.   Bridge Pose *(Setu Bhanda)*

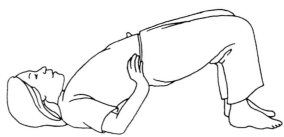

"Visualize in your mind where your stomach would be in the opposite of Bow Pose. What part of our body do we need to lie on now?"

"Lie down on your mat and pull your feet in so they are directly under your knees. Your toes should be pointed forward. Roll your shoulders back, so that there is a space under your neck to protect the bones in your neck, the cervical vertebrae. We have seven cervical vertebrae in our neck—guess how many a giraffe has in its neck? Giraffes have seven too!"

Bridge Pose

"Now press your arms into the floor and lift your hips off the floor, like a bridge over a river. You could push your hands up under your back to be a suspension bridge. Take two full breaths here, and then roll down to the mat, as if your vertebrae (the bones in your spine) are a string of pearls, rolling down one pearl at a time. Let's make another bridge, this time interlacing our fingers under our backs and resting them on the mat."

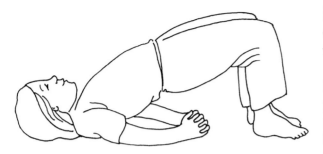

Bridge Pose

Note: There are students who may be comfortable doing a full backbend at this point.

Benefits: Bridge Pose is an energizing pose. It also stretches the abdominal muscles and strengthens the muscles in the back. It also stretches the muscles in the legs, which make it a good pose to do after sitting at a desk.

B: Theme 2: Math Yoga—Poses You Can Double

Math may not be a favorite subject of some students. Math yoga allows them to consider a fun way of doing math.

Suggestions for What to Say:

1.   Chair Pose to Hanging Bridge

a.   Chair Pose (*Utkatasana*)
"We may not have a chair, but let's take a seat anyway."
"Let's stand in Mountain Pose (Tadasana) with our feet about a foot apart. Roll your shoulders back and take a deep breath in through your nose. Stretch your arms out in front of you and pretend you are holding on to a bar. Now as you breathe out, begin to sit down. Do you feel how your weight shifts to your heels? See if you can sit a little bit more. Stay here for two breaths and then breathe yourself back up to Mountain Pose. Let's do that again. If you would like the challenge of a balance, try to lift your heels off the floor as you sit in your chair."

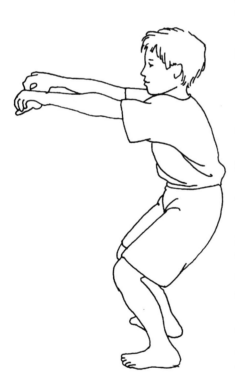

Chair Pose

Benefits: Chair Pose builds strength in the legs, arms, and the abdominal area (core).

b.   Hanging Bridge

"Picture in your mind how it would look if we doubled that pose."

"Let's practice all breathing in and out together. Find someone who is about your size. Reach toward each other and wrap your hands around the other person's wrists. At the same time, both take a deep breath in and then let the breath out. Let's do this again."

"Now, slowly bend toward each other as you each lean back, keeping your legs straight. Remember to breathe as you stretch your shoulders. After two breaths here, bend your knees at the same time and sit back. After two more breaths, each come down to a squat. Now slowly rise back up to the starting position. Let's try this again, remembering to breath in and out together."

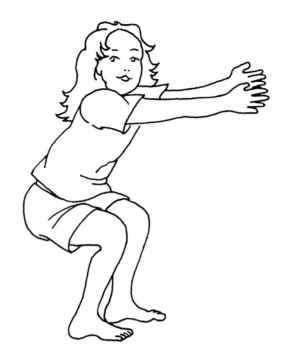

Chair Pose

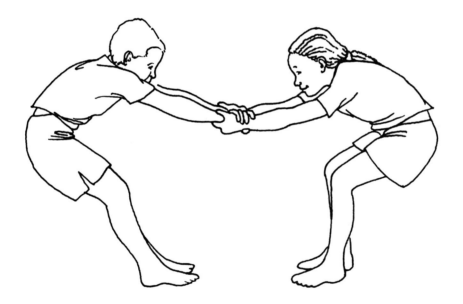

Hanging Bridge

Benefits: In addition to the benefits of Chair Pose, Hanging Bridge teaches awareness of breathing and cooperation.

2.   Boat Pose to Double Boat Pose
a.   Boat Pose (*Navasana*)

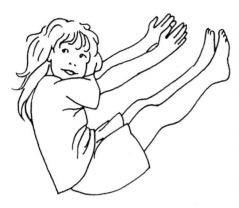

Boat Pose

"We are going to be a boat with a deep "V" shaped bottom. Imagine you are on a calm, peaceful lake. What do you see around you?"

"Sit with your legs out in front of you. Slowly bend your knees and lift your feet off the mat. You can wrap your arms around the backs of your legs so you can balance on your seat! When you extend your arms out does the boat start to rock? If it feels good, you can straighten your legs so your body is in a "V" shape, like the hull of a boat. How can you make your body calm and peaceful, just like the lake you imagine you are in? Maybe you want to bend your knees and hold your legs to calm the boat. Practice yoga by listening to your body."

Benefits: Boat Pose builds strength in the abdominal muscles. It is also a great pose for practicing balance, which means it also builds concentration!

b.   Double Boat Pose

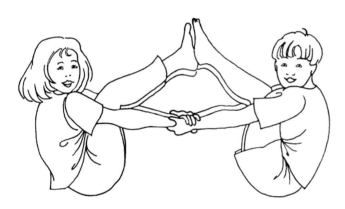

Double Boat Pose

"Picture in your mind how this pose would look if you doubled it. Let's see if we can do it."

"Find someone who has legs about the same length as yours. Sit facing each other, with your knees bent and feet flat on the mat. With your arms on the outside of your legs, grab hands so that your fingers are wrapped around each other's wrists. Now slowly raise one leg so that the soles of your feet touch. Straighten the legs up, just like in boat pose. Now do the same thing with the other legs, so that both of your legs are raised. Breathe together for three breaths. Come down, shake out your legs, and double your boat again."

Benefits: Adding to the benefits of Boat Pose, Double Boat Pose builds confidence in others, while it provides a superb shoulder stretch. It also shows kids how fun yoga can be.

3.   Crescent Moon to Double Crescent Moon

a.   Crescent Moon

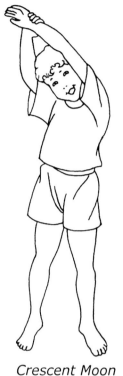

"Does anyone know what phase the moon is in now? Maybe you can look outside tonight. What does a crescent moon look like?"

"Let's start in Mountain Pose, with our arms down at our sides. As you slowly take a breath in, raise your arms toward the moon, reaching from your feet to the tips of your fingers. Imagine someone leaning down from a cloud and gently pulling you up. Take another inhale through your nose and put your hands together, with the index finger pointing up and the fingers interlaced. As you breathe out, reach to the right side and make a crescent moon. Breathe back to center and slowly bend to the other side. Let's do that again."

Benefits: Crescent Moon Pose is an energizing pose. It stretches the sides of your body (a lateral stretch) and the spine. It also builds strength in the abdominal area (core).

b.   Double Crescent Moon

Crescent Moon

"Imagine how Crescent Moon would look if we doubled it."

"Find someone about your height. Stand about three or four feet away from them. Each of you spread your feet so that your inside feet touch. Now bend toward each other and allow your inside arms to drop down, while your outside arms sweep up to meet over your heads. After you flow to one side twice, switch places so that your other side gets to be a crescent moon too."

Benefits: Adding to the benefits of Crescent Moon, this pose builds trust and confidence.

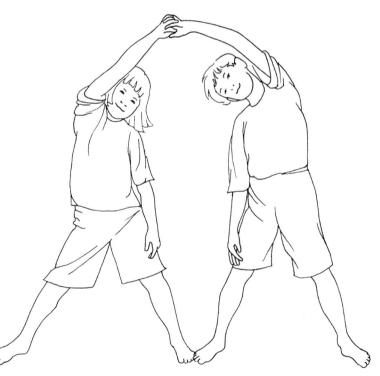

Double Crescent Moon

4.   Butterfly Pose to Kaleidoscope of Butterflies
a.   Butterfly Pose *(Baddha Konasana)*

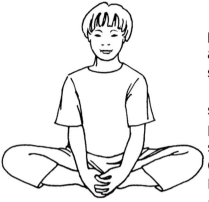

Butterfly Pose

"Picture a special place you would like to be a butterfly. Imagine how it smells and sounds."

"Let's be butterflies by sitting with straight spines and pulling our legs in so that the soles of our own feet touch. Our legs become flapping butterfly wings as we gently raise and lower our knees. I am flying to a rainforest—where would you like to fly?"

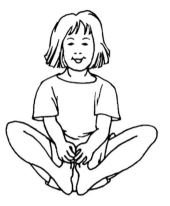

Butterfly Pose

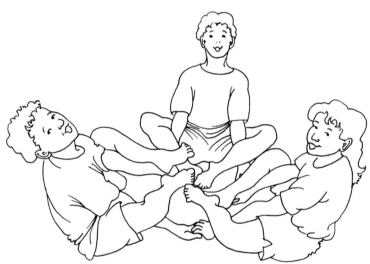

Kaleidoscope of Butterflies

b. Kaleidoscope of Butterflies Pose

"Have you ever seen a group of butterflies on some flowers or resting in a tree? Let's see if our group can make a group of colorful butterflies. Do you know what a group of butterflies is called? A kaleidoscope."

"Let's sit in a big circle with our knees almost touching. As we gently flap our butterfly wings, let's go around the circle and tell where we would like to fly. Now close your eyes and visualize a new place to fly!"

Note: You can reach your arms under your "folded wings" to grasp the hands of the person on either side. Then all together, have everyone try to balance on their seats! This quickly becomes a group favorite.

Benefits: This pose adds the benefits of working as a group and developing the ability to visualize desirable destinations.

5.   Half Forward Bend to Legs Up in the Air
a.   Half Forward Bend (*Ardha Uttanasana*)

"Pick a partner who is about your height. How can you make your body into half of a square with your feet on the floor?"

"Bend over so that your arms are next to your ears, your fingers are pointing straight toward the wall in front of you."

Benefits: This pose allows for a deep stretch in the back and hamstrings.

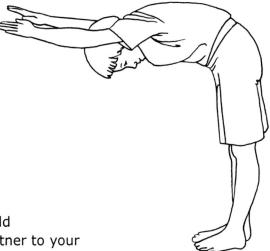

Half Forward Bend

b.   Legs Up in The Air

"How could we add your partner to your Forward Bend to complete the square?"

"What if the person lies on her back and puts her legs up in the air? Together you have made the square!

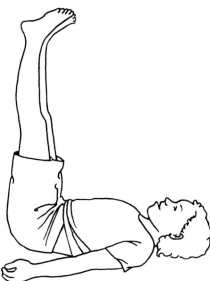

Legs Up in the Air

Breathe in together, and then breathe out together. Take three deep breaths here. Now switch places."

Note: You can do this "square" pose with or without a wall.

Benefits: This restorative pose helps to relieve tension in the body. Doing it as a double pose builds cooperation and an awareness of breathing.

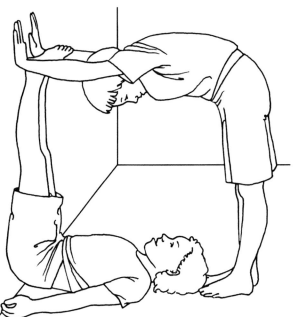

Making a Square

C: Theme 3: Poses that Melt

This section offers a series of flowing poses, called a *vinyasa*. "Vin" means "wind" in *Sanskrit*. Doing the poses in a flow keeps the students actively engaged as they think about what could come next. It is a fun sequence to do as the winter snows melt or as the summer heat melts popsicles.

Suggestions For What to Say:

1.   Downward Facing Dog to Plank to Upward Facing Dog
a.   Downward Facing Dog (*Adho Mukha Svanasana*)

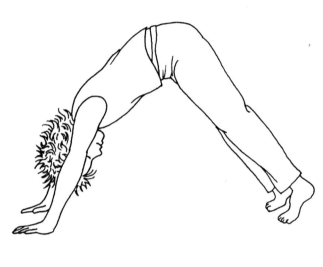

Down Dog

"Dogs like to stretch their muscles. It must feel good because they do this pose a lot. Let's try a pose we call Downward Facing Dog. Maybe you can think about what a dog you know does after he wakes up from a nap."

"Let's stretch our shoulders by pushing back from our hands and knees until our bottoms are flying high. Extra blood is going to your brain as your head hangs down and helps to lengthen your spine. Move your heels up and down as though you were pedaling a bike. Stay here for two breaths."

Benefits: Downward Facing Dog is a wonderful balancing pose—stretching down the backs of the legs and lifting up out of the back.

b.   Plank Pose

"Imagine the sun warming and relaxing your back as you melt by lowering your hips and moving your shoulders over your hands. Your toes are still curled under as your arms and legs hold your back off the floor."

Benefits: Plank Pose builds strength in the arms, abdomen, shoulders, and wrists. The pose also helps to lengthen the spine.

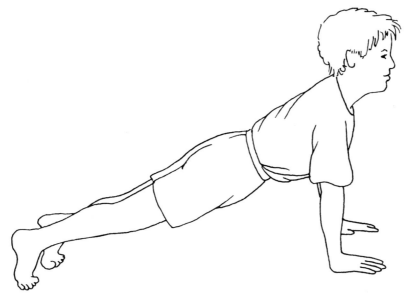

Plank Pose

c.   Upward Facing Dog (*Urdhva Mukha Svanasana*)

"Now breathe
out and melt a bit
more so that the tops
of your feet and legs
are resting on the floor.
Your arms are still
holding your hips off
the floor. Take several
full breaths here."

"Now finish
melting into a puddle—
you can even rest your
head on your arms.
Breathe!"

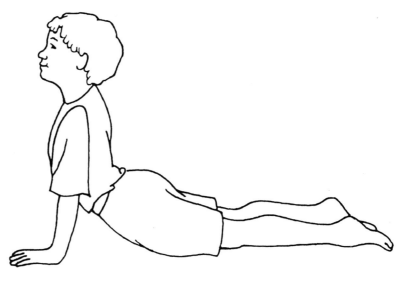

Upward Facing Dog

Note: Kids may like to melt from Plank into
Cobra (an easier pose), resting their hips on
the floor too. (Page 70)

**Benefits: Upward Facing Dog stretches the abdomen. It
strengthens the spine and arms. It also massages the
abdominal organs.**

2.   Mountain to Chair to Praying Mantis

a.   Mountain Pose (*Tadasana*)

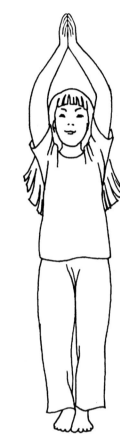

"Mountains are strong rocks that have been pushed out the earth. We are going to stand like tall strong mountains."

"Close your eyes and gently move back and forth on your feet until you feel balanced and strong, as if your feet are part of the rocky earth. Now breathe your hands up and reach for high into the azure blue sky."

Benefits: Doing Mountain Pose in this way helps develop a sense of balance and visualization.

b.   Chair Pose (*Utkatasana*)

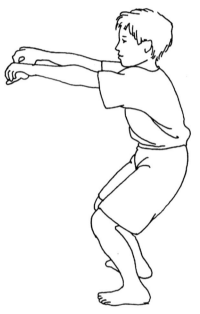

"Now let's take a seat by melting down into a chair. Even though we don't have a chair, we can pretend our bodies are chairs."

"Stretch your arms out in front of you and pretend you are holding on to a bar. Take a deep breath in through you nose, and as you start to breathe out, begin to sit down. Can you feel how your weight shifts to your heels? See if you can rest in your chair for another breath."

Mountain Pose

Chair Pose

Benefits: Chair Pose builds strength in your legs, legs, and abdominal area (core).

Chair Pose

c.   Praying Mantis

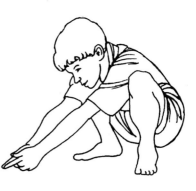

"Imagine that hot sun relaxing our muscles, melting us even more. Let's see where our breath takes us."

"Let your knees melt open to the side as you breathe yourself down into a squat. Now clasp your hands as you lean forward and point them toward the floor. Stretch your arms forward, like a praying mantis reaching for its food. Take three breaths here. Now let's go back up to Mountain Pose and melt down again."

Praying Mantis

Benefits: Praying Mantis opens the hips and shoulders. It also develops balance.

3.   Tree Pose to Bush Pose to Child's Pose
a.   Tree Pose (*Vrksasana*)

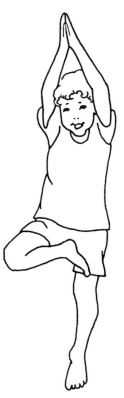

"Who can you think of a really tall tree? Did you know that a redwood tree can grow to over 300 feet? And some trees only grow to about 5 feet. What is your favorite kind of tree? Just as there are many kinds of trees, there are many ways to do Tree Pose. You can find the one that is right for your body today."

"Stand in Mountain Pose. Rock gently back and forth on your feet to find your balance point in the middle. Put all your weight in your right foot. Find a *drishti* or focus point, at eye level that is not moving. Now lift your left foot and rest it by your ankle, press it into your leg—either at your calf, above your knee, or high up on your thigh (not on your knee!)."

"Think of your foot and your standing leg having a conversation—each one is active and pressing the other back. It makes a strong post on which you can stand. Place your hands together in Prayer Pose at your chest. Slowly inhale through your nose as your hands reach up toward the sky. Can you use your arms to make yourself into a redwood tree? A maple tree with a round crown of branches? An aspen tree with leaves fluttering in the wind? How could we work together to make a forest?"

"Did you know that a grove of aspen trees is the largest living organism on the planet? One grove can be all one tree connected by underground roots!"

Note: Some people like the challenge of focusing on something that *is* moving or closing their eyes.

Tree Pose

Benefits: Tree pose helps develop focus and concentration. It builds balance and leg strength.

b.   Bush Pose

"Bushes are woody plants that do not grow as tall as trees. Let's melt into a bush. Move the foot of your bent leg across the top of your standing leg. Melt down as you slowly bend your standing leg. Melt as far as you can, and then release your leg to the floor and sit on your knees."

Benefits: Bush pose helps builds balance, confidence, and leg strength.

c.   Child's Pose *(Balasana)*

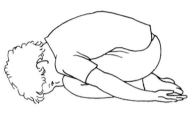

Child's Pose

"Let's keep melting into Child's Pose. Let your back and head melt down to rest on the floor. Your bottom is sitting on your feet. Your hands can rest by your heels or your arms can stretch out over your head. Take three easy breaths here. Then we will grow into Tree Pose and melt again, as though it is a very hot day.

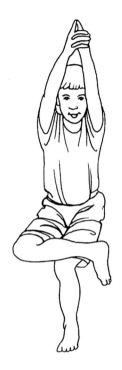

Bush Pose

Benefits: Child's Pose is a gentle lower backstretch. It also is a resting pose, allowing the body time to absorb the benefits of the previous pose.

4.   Half Shoulderstand to Boat Pose to Seastar Pose
a.   Half Shoulderstand (*Ardha Sarvangasana*)

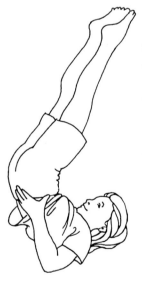

"Usually we stand on our feet, but in the last pose we stood on our knees. What other parts of the body could we stand on? Let's see if we can stand on our upper back."
"Watch me do this pose first. It is important not to turn your head in this pose because you could really hurt your neck. First, lie flat on your mat. Roll your shoulders up toward your ears and then roll them back into the mat. Tilt your chin up so your hand will fit under your neck. Place your hands on the lower part of your back, so you can press your elbows into the mat and lift up. Breathe! Use your arms to push your legs up into the air. Only go up as far as it feels good."

Caution: It is best to only do Half Shoulderstand. Full Shoulderstand without proper preparation and individual supervision can cause neck injuries.

Half Shoulderstand

Benefits: Shoulderstand calms the body. It allows the lungs to open. As the blood drains from the feet, circulation to the brain is increased.

b.   Boat Pose (*Navasana*)

"As you breathe out, allow yourself to slowly melt to the floor, but leave your legs up. Now sit up so that you are balancing on your bottom. Hold your arms out for balance. Remember, you can bend your knees and wrap your arms around the backs of your legs if that feels better. Listen to your body."

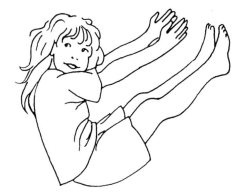

Benefits: Boat Pose builds strength in the abdominal muscles. It is also a great pose for practicing balance, which means it also builds concentration!

Boat Pose

c.   Seastar Pose

"Imagine what would happen to Boat Pose if you just let your arms and legs melt down to the floor. Take a deep breath in through your nose and as you release the breath, melt down to the earth. Allow your arms and legs to point out, so your seastar has five rays. What is the fifth ray? (the head). Relax here for a few breaths. Then let's find Half Shoulderstand and melt again, as slowly as ice melting in the spring."

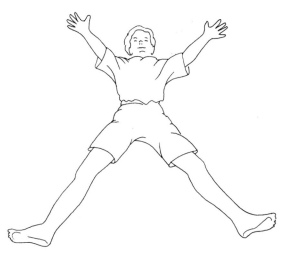

Seastar Pose

Benefits: Seastar Pose done on the floor gives a gentle stretch to the arms and legs. As a resting pose, it gives time for the body to absorb the benefits of the previous pose.

D. Theme 4: Poses You Can Do In Line and Those You Cannot!

There are yoga poses that can make waiting in a line more fun. After you do this theme once, kids will continue to think of poses to add.

Suggestions for What to Say:

1.   Poses to Do in Line
a.   Mountain Pose (*Tadasana*)

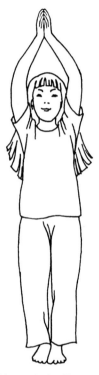

Mountain Pose

"Stand like a tall mountain. Find a comfortable place for your feet and gently rock back and forth to find the point where you feel balanced and strong, the base of a mountain. Lift your toes, find your balance, and then let your toes relax back onto the mat. Roll your shoulders back, keep your eyes looking forward. Now breathe your hands up and reach for the clouds.

Benefits: Mountain Pose is a standing pose that helps with balance and good posture.

b.   Tree Pose (*Vrsksasana*)

"Can you be like a tree while standing in line?"

"Stand in Mountain Pose and think of your favorite tree. Rock gently back and forth on your feet to find your balance point in the middle. Put all your weight in your right foot. Find a *drishti* point, a point at eye level that is not moving, on which to focus. (A challenge is to focus on something that is moving!) Now lift your left foot and either rest it by your ankle or press it into your leg—either at your calf, above your knee, or high up on your thigh (not on your knee!) Think of your foot and your standing leg having a conversation—each one is active and pressing the other back. Your right leg makes a strong post on which you can stand. Place your hands together in prayer pose at your chest."

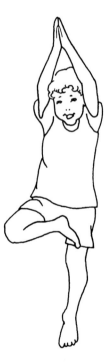

Tree Pose

Benefits: Tree Pose helps develop focus and concentration. It builds balance and leg strength.

c.   King Dancer or Lord of the Dance Pose (*Natarajasana*)

"Do you think it would be fun
to dance in line? Let's try King Dancer
or Lord of the Dance Pose."

"Start in Mountain Pose, solid
and strong like a granite mountain.
Now lift your left foot and reach
around with your left hand to grab
your ankle or the top of your foot.
Breathe in and raise your right hand
out in front of you for balance. As
you breathe out, slowly bend forward
from the waist and kick your back
leg into your hand. How far you bend
depends on your body and on how
many people are in line!"

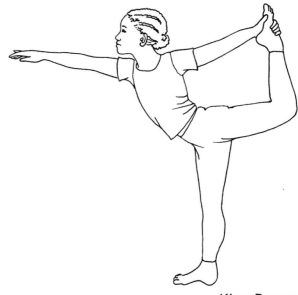

King Dancer

**Benefits: King Dancer Pose helps develop focus, balance,
and concentration. It stretches the legs and abdomen.**

2.   And Those You Cannot Do in Line
a.   Pretzel Pose (*Ardha Matsyendrasana*)

"Is sitting down and twisting like a pretzel a good pose for
doing in a line? Let's try so you can decide."

"Sit with your legs stretched out in front of
you. Draw your right leg in so that the foot rests next
to the left thigh. Pick up the right foot and place it
on the other side of your left leg. Now swing your
left foot in toward your bottom. Place your left hand
on your right knee and gently twist to the right,
looking over your right shoulder. Remember to keep
your spine tall. If you want, you can make more of
a pretzel wrap by wrapping your right hand around
your back. On your next breath out, see if you can
twist a little bit more. Now slowly unwind. Yoga is
about keeping things in balance, so we need to make
a pretzel on the other side now. Why do you think
this might not a good pose to do in a line?"

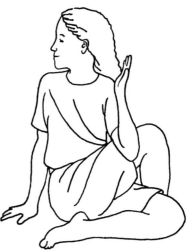

Pretzel Pose

**Benefits: Twists help increase flexibility of the spine. They also
"squeeze" out the internal organs like wringing a sponge. After
the twist, the organs are infused with a fresh supply of blood.**

b.   Crow Pose (*Kakasana*)

"Do you think balancing on your hands is a good pose for doing in a line? After we do Crow Pose, see what you think. The crow is an intelligent, strong bird with large wings."

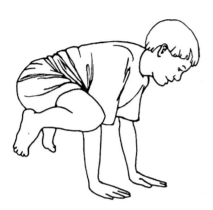

"Squat down with your feet under your hips. Lean forward and tuck the top part of your arms between your legs. Now press your arms out while you press your knees against your arms! Pull in your belly, or core, muscles—now slowly lean forward on your hands. Come up to your tiptoes, and, if you can, lift one leg off the floor. Don't lift your hips too high, or you will become a diving bird! Your legs are balancing on your bent arms—which is why this pose is called an arm balance. If your body wants to try, lift both feet off the mat while balancing on your arms. Slowly come down and try it again. Often a pose is easier to do the second time around."

Crow Pose

Benefits: Crow Pose develops balance, focus, and strength of purpose.

c.   Bow 'n Arrow Pose

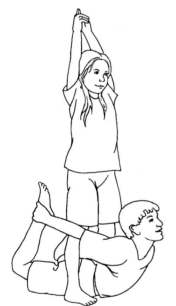

"Do you think lying on your belly is good to do in a line? Would you do it if someone were standing over you with her arms pointed to the sky? Let's do Bow'n Arrow Pose and see what you think."

"Find someone to be your partner. One person will lie on his stomach and reach back with his left hand and grab his left foot. He will then reach back with his right hand and grab his right foot. He can arch his back up as he kicks back into his hands, so his body goes up like a bow. The other person, the 'arrow', stands with her feet on either side of the 'bow's' hips, legs to the inside of the 'bow's' arms. The 'arrow' stands with her fingers interlaced, arms straight over her head, like an arrow ready to shoot. Listen for each other's breath and breathe together—a deep breath in through the nose and a long, slow breath out. Try breathing together for 4 breaths and then switch spots."

Bow'n Arrow Pose

Benefits: Bow Pose stretches the abdominals and the shoulders. Arrow Pose builds balance and lengthens the spine. Doing the pose with a partner builds cooperative skills.

E.   Theme 5: Poses That Make You Feel Powerful

One of the many benefits of yoga is that it can build inner strength of purpose as well as develop muscles. Standing poses can help kids feel physically stronger and raise their confidence.

Suggestions for What to Say:

1.   Warrior 1 *(Virabhadrasana* 1)

"Warrior 1 is a pose named after a mythical warrior, Virabhadra, who is said to have a thousand heads, a thousand feet, and a thousand eyes. When you do this pose it helps you to feel strong without hurting anyone. What do you need to be strong to accomplish?"

"Stand sideways with your right leg toward the front of your mat. Place your feet about a leg-length apart and turn your toes in like a duck. You may want to quack three times! Now leave your left foot planted on the mat, and slowly turn your right toes toward the front, without moving your heel. Pretend you have a headlight on each hip and turn them to shine over your front foot. Breathe your arms up. Now bend your front knee (but make sure the knee does not go out over the toes because that will hurt the knee) and sink your hips down as far as it feels comfortable. Take a full breath and lift your arms toward the clouds. Flow back up to standing. Let's do this again."

Warrior 1

Benefits: Warrior 1 strengthens the legs and opens the chest. It improves balance and builds stamina and confidence.

2.   Warrior 2 (*Virabhadrasana* 2)

"Another type of warrior holds a large bow. You have to be confident and strong to use such a bow. Let's see how Warrior 2 makes us feel."

"With your feet in the same position as in Warrior 1, turn the headlights on your hips so they now face the left side of the room. Breathe your arms up so they extend in a single line across your back. Turn your head and look out over your right middle finger, as if you were about to shoot an arrow from a bow. On you next exhale, bend your right knee and let your hips sink down. Now

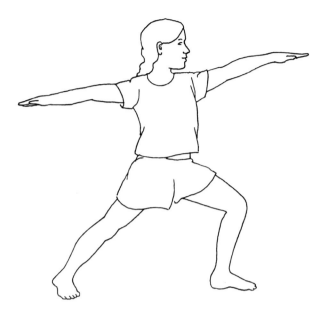

lower your arms as you straighten your leg and come back up. Then raise your arms and let your hips melt down again. Let's do this three times. Now let's rest in Child's Pose for five long breaths."

Benefits: Warrior 2 strengthens the legs and opens the chest. It improves balance and builds stamina and confidence.

Warrior 2

3.   Rocket Pose 1 *(Parsvakonasana)*

"What do you think of when you think of a rocket? I think a rocket packs a lot of power. Let's get our bodies set up for Rocket Pose and see how strong we feel."

"Find Warrior 2 again with your right leg forward. Bend and rest your right arm on the top of your right thigh. On *your* next breath in, sweep your left arm over your head, next to your ear. If someone had a ruler, could they draw a line from the tip of your left hand to the heel of your left foot? Think of a rocket blasting out of your arm. Breathe in two long breaths. Come down out of the pose, and then let's do it once more. This time bend your elbow and rest your arm on top of your leg."

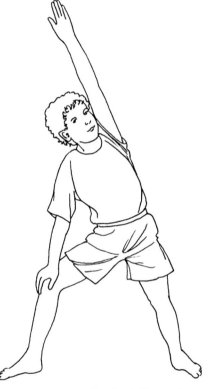

Rocket Pose 1

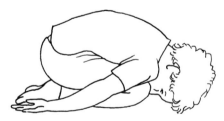

Child's Pose

"Let's use this opportunity to listen to our bodies. We will rest in Child's Pose for a few breaths."

Benefits: Rocket Pose gives the body an intense side stretch. It also opens the chest.

4.   Warrior 3 (*Virabhadrasana* 3) or "T" Pose

"Would you like to try the third Warrior Pose so you know another way to build your own power? Why would you like to be stronger?"

"Stand in Mountain Pose, with your arms reaching over your head. Shift all your weight onto your right foot. Step your left leg back so the toes touch the mat. Take a deep breath in and, as you breathe out, bend forward from the waist so that your arms go out like a "T". If your body would like, you may lift your back leg, so your whole body becomes the letter "T". Breathe your leg and arms down. Let's do it one more time."

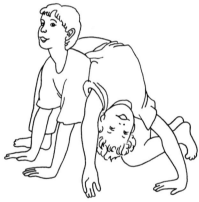

Warrior 3

Note: Kids can lean toward a friend and rest their arms on the friend's shoulders to feel the full stretch. A challenge is to begin in Warrior 1 and move into Warrior 3.

Benefits: Warrior 3 strengthens the legs and arms. It improves balance and builds stamina and confidence.

5.   Waterfall Pose

"Sometimes it makes you feel strong and powerful to have support from a friend. Giving support or help to a friend can make us feel strong too! Find someone about your size to be a friend."

"One person gets on their hands and knees. They are the rock over which the water is going to flow. The second person can stand on her knees, back toward the "rock", and slowly slide her back over the "rock" in a supported backbend. Do NOT sit on the person's back. Only your backs should be touching. Breathe in and then out at the same time your friend does. Do this three times. Then we will switch spots."

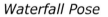

Waterfall Pose

Note: Heavier students should not lie over smaller students. Perhaps they can be a waterfall over you. Make sure the kids are paired according to approximate size and weight.

Benefits: This builds back strength, awareness of breathing, and cooperation. It is also a gentle way to move the spine.

F.   Theme 6: Poses that Flow

This section offers another way to do a *vinyasa*, or a series of poses that flow. Use the breath to connect the pose—meaning you should keep breathing as you move into the next pose. Doing a flow helps people build focus as they think about what is coming next.

Suggestions for What to Say:

1.   Warrior 1 to Warrior 2 to Reverse Warrior 2
a.   Warrior 1 (Virabhadrasana 1)

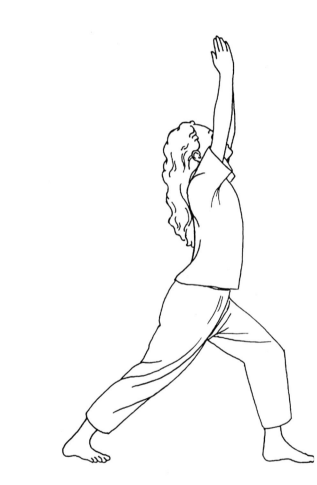

Warrior 1

"The Warrior poses are about being strong. You can be strong without hurting someone. Close your eyes and think about something that you need to have courage or feel strong to do. Now open your eyes so that we can be warriors."

"Strengthen your legs by stepping your feet apart, with your right foot toward the front of the mat. Turn your toes in a little, and then point your right foot toward the front. Feel your chest grow stronger, ready to receive your deep breath, as you turn your hips to face over your front foot. Breathe your arms over your head. Feel the muscles in your legs grow stronger as you slowly bend your right knee and take a deep breath."

Note: Make sure the front knee does not extend over the front foot, as this may injure the knee.

Benefits: Warrior 1 gives kids a sense of empowerment without them hurting anyone.

b.   Warrior 2 (*Virabhadrasana* 2)

"Keeping your legs in the same position, turn the headlights on your hips so they face the side of the room. Breathe your arms down so they extend in a single line across your back. Turn your head and look out over your right middle finger, as if you were about to shoot arrow from a bow. On *your* next exhale, bend your right knee and let your hips melt down. Now we are going to flow like a river into Reverse Warrior 2."

Benefits: Warrior 2 strengthens the legs and opens the chest. It improves balance and builds stamina and confidence.

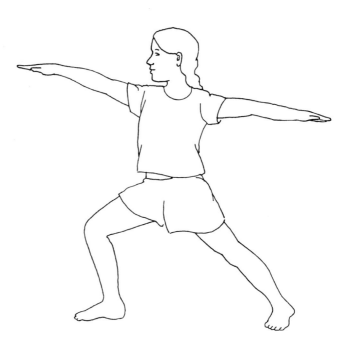

Warrior 2

c.   Reverse Warrior 2

"Slide your left hand down the back of your back (left) leg. On *your* next breath in, sweep your right hand in an arc over your head, just like you are a crescent moon. Let's put the whole thing in reverse, to flow back to Warrior 1. Can we flow one more time since our bodies know where we are going?"

Benefits: Reverse Warrior 2 strengthens the legs and opens the side of the body. It improves balance and builds stamina and confidence.

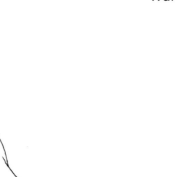

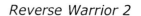

Reverse Warrior 2

2.   Gate Pose to Reverse Gate Pose
a.   Gate Pose (*Parighasana*)

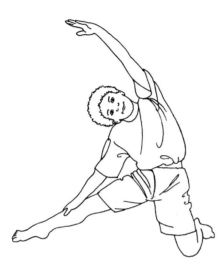

Gate Pose

"Do you know a place with a gate? When you open it, where can you go? Gates are about opening—so let's do Gate Pose and open our bodies to breathing more easily. Close your eyes and imagine a gate opening into a place that is special to you."

"Stand on your knees, and roll you shoulders back to create space for your lungs to expand. Put one hand on your chest and take a deep breath. Can you feel how more air can go into the space you just created? Open your right leg out to the side, just like opening a book. You can either keep your knee bent or for more of a challenge, straighten the leg as you extend it. As you take your next inhale, sweep your left arm into an arc over your head. Your right arm can move down to your right leg or to the floor. Remember to breathe as you move."

Benefits: Gate Pose provides a deep stretch for the side of the body, the intercostal muscles. When these muscles are tight, the rib cage is constricted, so we cannot breathe as deeply.

b.   Reverse Gate Pose

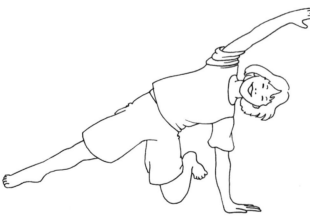

Reverse Gate Pose

"Some gates swing in and some gates swing out. Let's swing to the other side and make even more space for breathing. Close your eyes and imagine a new place into which your gate opens. Perhaps it opens onto a sandy beach in the summer or into a field of wildflowers in the spring."

"Sweep your left hand back to rest on the floor on your left side. Straighten your right leg and push your hips up toward the sky. Now sweep your right arm in an arc over your head. Take two deep breaths. Now let's sweep back to Gate Pose and try that again."

Benefits: Reverse Gate Pose provides a deep stretch for the other side of the body. Doing Gate Pose and Reverse Gate Pose together creates room in the chest for deeper breathing.

3. Downward Facing Dog to Raised Mountain to Knee-to-Nose Pose
a. Downward Facing Dog

"How many of you have dogs?
You may have seen your dog do this
next pose after he wakes up from a nap.
This is why it is called Downward Facing
Dog or Down Dog."

"Get on your hands and knees
with a flat back with your hands under
your shoulders. Yawn as though you are
just waking up. Now you need to stretch,
so curl your toes under and push your
hips up. Press one heel down and then
the other, as though you are pedaling on
a bike. Now straighten your legs and push
your heels down toward the floor. Take
a deep breath and enjoy the stretch, just
like dogs do!"

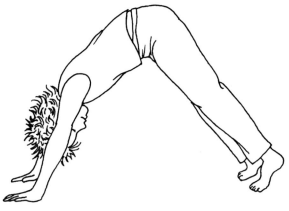

Down Dog

**Benefits: Down Dog is a great shoulder stretch. It also helps
you to lengthen your spine and stretch the hamstring and calf
muscles in the backs of your legs. It also allows extra blood to
go to the head, bringing oxygen and nutrients to the brain.**

b. Raised Mountain Pose

"Now how could we make this
pose tall like a mountain, only moving
one part of our body? How could we
become taller by using our legs?"

"Raise your right let up toward
the sky. I think we all look a lot taller!
Take a breath here and lower your
leg. Find your Down Dog again. Now
breathe in and raise your left leg to
make another mountain. Breathe
your leg down, and we can all meet in
Down Dog."

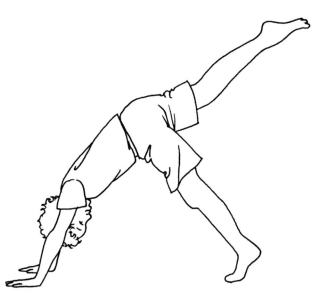

Raised Mountain Pose

**Benefits: Raised Mountain has all
the benefits of Downward Facing Dog. It also opens
the hip muscles, stimulates the immune system by
moving the lymph, and improves circulation.**

c.   Raised Mountain to Nose-to-Knee Pose

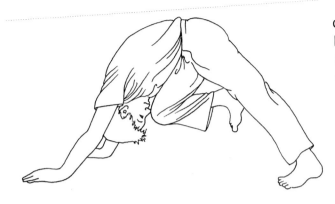

Raised Mountian Nose-to-Knee

"If your body would like, come down on your knees. Or, if your body wants to be in a full, refreshing stretch, stay in Down Dog. Either way, let's see how our legs can flow like a stream in spring."

"Whichever pose you are starting from, look down toward your belly button as you push your breath out and bring your knee in to touch your nose. Then let the right leg flow back to Down Dog (or let your knee go back to the floor. Do the same thing three more times on this side. Let's flow on the left side now."

Benefits: Knee-to-Nose builds arm strength, flexibility in the spine, and coordination. Giving people choices reinforces that yoga is about listening to your body.

4.   Seesaw

"How many people does it take to play on a seesaw? Shall we try to make a seesaw out of people?"

"Find a partner who has legs about the same length as yours. Sit facing her, with your knees bent and feet flat on the mat. With your arms on the outside of your bent legs, grab hands so that your fingers are wrapped around the other person's wrists. Now slowly raise one leg so that the sole of your foot touches the sole of her foot. Slowly raise and straighten your legs toward the sky, just like in Boat Pose. Now do the other leg, so that both of your legs are pointing straight up. As you both breathe in, rock slightly

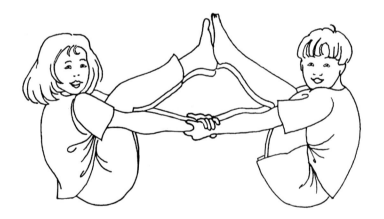

Seesaw

toward one person, then as you both breathe out rock back toward the other. Can you breathe together while you balance on your bottom."

Note: After the kids are familiar with this pose, begin with the fun "Seesaw Balance" game found on page 117.

Benefits: Breathing with a partner in a flowing pose develops a sense of one's own breathing and moving with the breath. The pose strengthens the abdominal and leg muscles, and provides a good shoulder stretch. It also shows kids how fun yoga can be, while building skills of balance and cooperation.

5.   Waterfall Pose

"How can water flow in beautiful ways? Have you ever sat near a waterfall and listened? Shall we make a waterfall?"

"Choose a partner who is about your size. One person gets down in flat back, on their hands and knees. They are the rock over which the water is going to flow. The second person can stand on her knees, back toward the 'rock', and slowly slide her back over the 'rock' in a supported backbend. Only your backs should be touching— do NOT sit on the person's back. Can you make the waterfall higher by both breathing in together? After three breaths, you can switch spots."

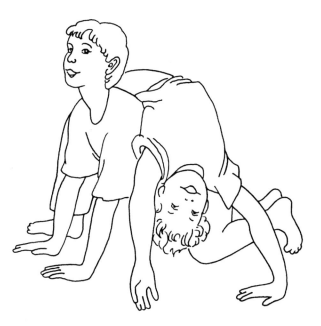

Waterfall Pose

Note: Perhaps you can allow heavier students to do the pose with you to prevent anyone from getting hurt! Make sure the kids are paired by size.

Benefits: This pose builds back strength, an awareness of breathing, and a feeling of cooperation.

G.   Theme 7: Poses that Grow

This section offers another way to do a *vinyasa*, or a series of poses that flow. The section gives kids a chance to consider how poses can evolve. And since kids are still growing, these flows may cause them to wonder what they might grow into next.

Suggestions for What to Say:

1.   Child's Pose into Cobra into Upward Facing Dog into Mountain Pose Child's Pose (*Balasana*)

a.   Child's Pose

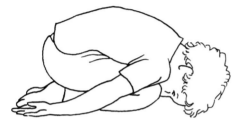

"Have many of you have grown since you were little kids? Do you think you can make Child's Pose grow? Let's try it together."

"Sit back on your heels, round your back, and slowly lower your head and chest to the floor. You are now a child again."

Child's Pose

Note: It can be fun to do this pose facing a friend. Each person sits at different ends of the same mat. Keep in mind they will need room to stretch out in the following poses.

Benefits: Child's Pose is a resting pose that provides a gentle backstretch, while it releases the muscles in the lower back.

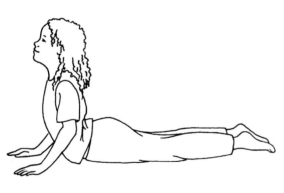

b.   Cobra Pose (*Bhujangasana*)

"People stretch as we grow, so let's pull ourselves forward and stretch our on our mats. Put your hands under your shoulders and slowly lift your back like a snake. Hiss like a cobra. Remember that snakes do not have arms, so lift from your back. Can you keep the snake up even if you lift your hands off your mat? Roll your shoulder back to open your chest. Take a deep inhale and hiss again."

Cobra

Benefits: Cobra Pose helps keep the spine flexible, strengthens the lower back, and opens the chest.

c.   Upward Facing Dog or Updog (*Urdha Mukha Svanasana*)

"Now we can keep growing by rolling our toes under and pushing up on our hands. Now our chest and hips are off the ground. Keep your shoulders rolled toward your back so you can take a deep breath and fill your open chest with air. After a deep inhale, bark like a happy, growing dog."

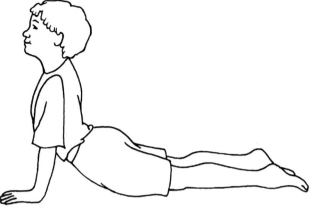

Upward Facing Dog

Benefits: Up Dog stimulates the kidneys and the adrenal glands. It strengthens the arms and the back.

d.   Mountain Pose (*Tadasana*)

"What pose would show us how much you actually have grown since you were a small child? Let's slowly roll our spines up to standing. Now breathe your arms up and point your fingers toward the sky. You have grown into a tall mountain. Let's try that again from Child's Pose."

Benefits: Mountain Pose is a standing pose that helps with balance and good posture. It lengthens the spine and opens the chest.

Mountain Pose

2. Squat into Forward Bend into Mountain Pose into Rooster Pose

a. Squat

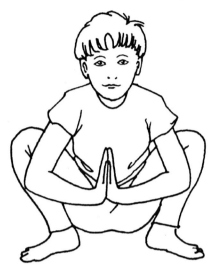

"How does a little guy look at the world? Let's get a kids' eye view of things."

"Sit in a squat, with your feet a comfortable distance apart. Let your knees fall open. Put your palms together resting your thumbs on your chest, and let your arms rest in front of your knees. How can we make this pose grow a little?"

Benefits: Squat Pose helps to open the hips, while stretching the feet and ankles. Sitting in a squat also improves balance and focus.

Squat

b. Forward Bend (*Uttanasana*)

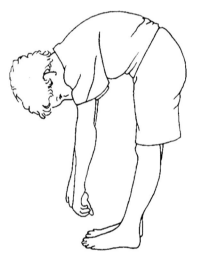

"Now grow a little by putting your hands out in front of you and slowly lifting your seat toward the sky into a Forward Bend. Keep your knees soft (bent) if that feels good. You look bigger already.

"Benefits: Forward Bend lengthens the spine. It can also stretch the legs muscles, but the focus of the pose is the backstretch.

Forward Bend

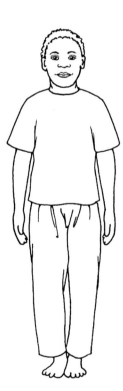

c. Mountain Pose (*Tadasana*)

"On your next breath in, keep your arms by your ears and slowly roll your spine up, breathing in to make yourself taller. Now you are seeing the world from your own view. Roll your shoulders back and take another breath in as you raise your arms high over your head. How could you make yourself even taller?"

Benefits: Doing Mountain Pose in this sequence helps kids to see that there are other ways of looking at things.

Mountain Pose

d.   Rooster Pose

"Keep your arms reaching toward the clouds and rise up
on your tiptoes. Feel as though someone is leaning down from a
cloud and gently pulling you up. Lower your heels, and then rise up
again. Keep your ankles moving toward each other as your rise up.
When you feel your calf muscles, reach up a bit higher! Come down
when your body needs to. Let's use our breath to grow one more
time."

**Benefits: Rooster Pose is a standing pose that helps with
balance and focus. It is also a good stretch for the calf muscles.**

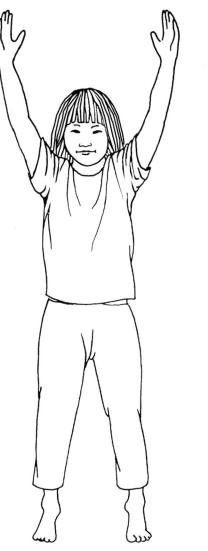

Rooster Pose

3. Child's Pose into Cat Pose into Down Dog
a. Child's Pose (*Balasana*)

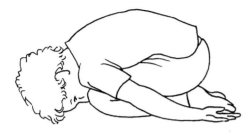

"Since we all started out as small children, let's go back to Child's Pose."

"Sit back on your heels. Let your back and head melt down to the earth, with your arms down by your side or out in front of you. Keep your back rounded like a turtle shell."

Child's Pose

Benefits: Child's Pose is a resting pose that provides a gentle backstretch, while it releases the muscles in the lower back.

b. Cat Pose

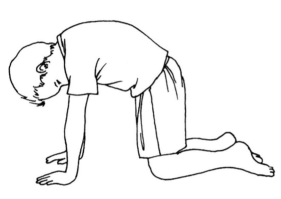

"Let's grow into our Cat Pose by pushing our backs up with the breath. Now take a deep breath, and as you breathe out, arch your back even more, dropping your head and hissing like a fierce cat. What are you hissing at?

Benefits: Cat Pose provides a gentle stretch to the spine and the back. It also is an easy way to draw awareness to moving with the breath.

Cat Pose

c. Downward Facing Dog (*Adho Mukha Svanasana*)

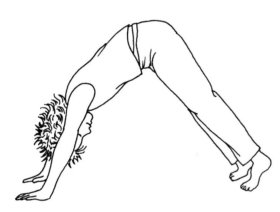

"Maybe the cat is hissing at the dog. Let's keep growing by curling our toes under and pushing our hips up into Down Dog. Remember to press down through your heels to really stretch the muscles in the backs of your legs. Can your dog bark back at the cat? Now let's find our Child's Pose and take four breaths here. Then we can start to grow again"

Benefits: Down Dog is a wonderful shoulder stretch. It also stretches out the back and the legs, while helping to build arm and shoulder strength.

Down Dog

4.   Pyramid Pose into Triangle into Warrior 2
a.   Pyramid Pose (*Parsvottanasana*)

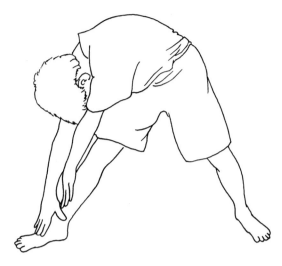

Pyramid Pose

"What is a pyramid shape? What are the pyramids in Egypt made from? Let's see if we can use yoga to move a pyramid we make."

"Stand sideways on your mat facing the left side of the room. Step your feet apart and turn your toes in like a duck. Let's quack 3 times.* Now turn the right foot so that it faces me toward the front of the room. Find your balance point by moving back and forth and adjusting your feet position. Now on your next breath in, raise your arms over your head. As you exhale, melt down over your front leg. Only bend as far as it feels good. You are shaped like a pyramid now. Breathe here for two breaths. Now let's move the pyramid by growing into the next pose."

Note: *By specifying the number of quacks, kids can have fun with the pose, but it will not get out of hand.

Benefits: Pyramid Pose is a strong stretch for the backs of the legs. It also improves balance and focus.

b.   Triangle Pose *(Trikonasana)*

"From your pyramid, put weight into your right hand resting on your leg (not your knee!) or the floor. Use your breath to sweep your arm up into Triangle Pose.

Benefits: Triangle Pose stretches the sides of the body and increases flexibility in the hips and spine.

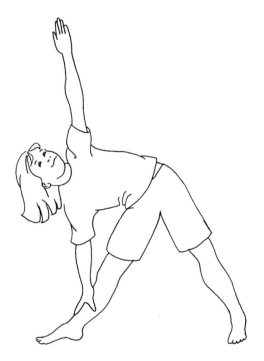

Triangle Pose

c.   Warrior 2 (Virabhadrasana 2)

"How could we grow taller from Triangle Pose? As if someone were standing behind you gently pulling on your left hand, rise up to standing. Keep both arms extended so that you have grown into Warrior 2."

"Turn the headlights on your hips so they both face the side of the room. Turn your head and look out over your right middle finger, as if you were about to shoot a bow and arrow. Now let's come down into Child's Pose and rest for four breaths before we grow again."

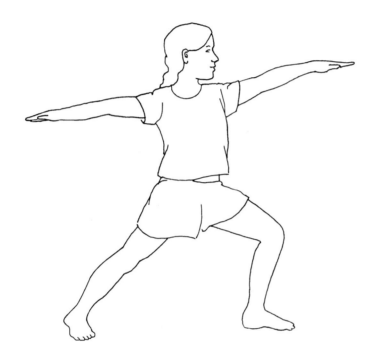

Warrior 2

Benefits: Doing poses in a flowing sequence shows the kids transitions can be a smooth and important part of the process. Warrior 2 strengthens the legs and opens the chest. It improves balance and builds stamina and confidence.

H.   Theme 8: Poses That Get Wet

In addition to the physical benefits of each of these poses, this theme allows kids another opportunity to practice visualization. They can add other poses to the section as they consider how those might get wet!

Suggestions for What to Say:

1.   Seastar

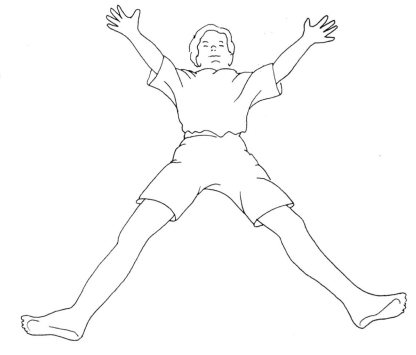

Seastar

"Seastars live on the ocean's edge. Many live in tide pools, areas that get wet when the tide comes in twice a day. Seastars have five rays that radiate out from their core, or central area. How can we be seastars?"

"Lie down and spread your arms and feet wide as you stretch to the tips of your fingers. Now stretch to the tips of your toes. Stretch your head away from your shoulders, so now you have the five arms (two legs, two arms, one head!) of a seastar. Close your eyes and wiggle your fingers and toes while you imagine the waves washing over you. Let's take a deep breath in and then slowly release the breath. Can you feel the ocean water lapping over your fingers and toes?"

Note: You can also do this pose standing.

Benefits: This pose energizes the body as it opens the chest, which allows for deeper breathing. It also offers a guided visualization practice.

2.   Frog (Bhekasana) to Leap Frog
a.   Frog Pose

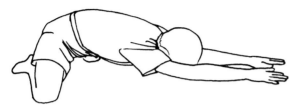

"Frogs have strong back legs for leaping. First let's stretch our hips, so we can be ready to jump."

"Get on your hands and knees so you look like a table. Then move each knee out to the side. On your next deep breath, as you breathe out, slowly sit back. Move back until your body tells you to stop. After two breaths, move back to your hands and knees and try it again.

Frog Pose

b.   Leap Frog

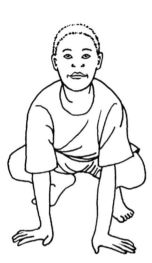

"To leap like a frog, squat down on the back of your mat. Your arms are inside your knees and your palms are on the floor. When your body feels like leaping, put your weight into your hands and allow your legs to straighten in a leap forward. Let's try this several times."

Benefits: Frog Pose is a great way to stretch the hips and the insides of the thighs. It is an energizing pose, so it is a nice way to perk up a practice.

3.   Swimmer 1 Pose

Leap Frog

"Where do you like to swim—in a river, a lake, the ocean, or a pool? Imagine being in your favorite spot for swimming while you lie on your belly and stretch your arms in front of you."

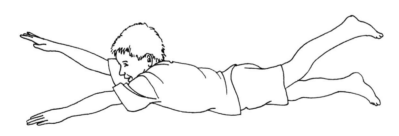

"As you take a breath in, raise your right arm and hold it there, and as you breathe out, raise your left leg. Hold them up for another breath. Slowly

Swimmer 1

release back to the floor. Now let's do the other side. Swimming is fun, so let's do this two more times. Imagine swimming in a new place or with new friends. Are you swimming in a race?"

Benefits: The pose builds strength in the core and lengthens the spine. It also exercises the visual imagination.

4.   Fish *(Matsyasana)*

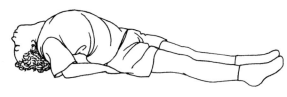

"How many of you have a favorite fish? In what kind of water does it live—salt water or fresh water?"

"Let's lie down on our backs and pull our legs up so that our feet are right under our knees. Pretend you have pockets on the back of your pants and slide your hands, palms facing the floor, into them. Even if you do have pockets, put your hands directly on the floor. As you breathe in, gently arch your back so the top of your head rolls back to the floor. Close your eyes and think about swimming with your favorite fish. After a few breaths, gently release your whole body to the floor as you breathe out. Let's do this one more time. After you release your head, hug your knees into your chest and rest."

Fish Pose

Benefits: Fish Pose gently increases the flexibility of the spine. It opens the chest and allows for deeper breathing.

5.   Rainbow Pose *(Vasisthasana)*

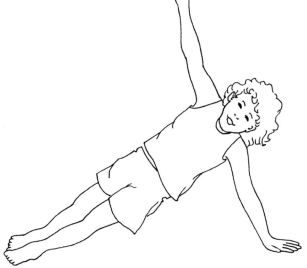

"Do you remember where you last saw a rainbow? Who knows the colors of a rainbow? (Red, orange, yellow, green, blue, indigo, violet) Let's see if you can be a rainbow and feel the sunlight shining through raindrops."

"First, move into Downward Facing Dog. Drop your right knee to the floor. Keep your left leg straight and roll over onto your bent right leg and the inside of your left foot. Use your right arm to hold you up, and breathe your left arm up toward the sky. Can you reach up a centimeter more to spread your rainbow out? Lift your hips up with you! Now close your eyes as you imagine that your body is made up of the colors of the rainbow."

Rainbow Pose

"If your body feels like a challenge today, straighten your right leg so that you are balancing on the outside of your right foot with the inside of your left foot stacked on top of it!"

Benefits: Rainbow pose improves balance and concentration. It also builds arm strength and stretches the leg muscles.

I.   Theme 9: Things You Find Outside

You can do yoga anywhere, and this theme brings together some poses named after things we find outside. It also gives kids the opportunity to make up their own poses to fit the theme. And remember that in nice weather, it is fun to do these poses out-of-doors.

Suggestions for What to Say:

1.   Praying Mantis

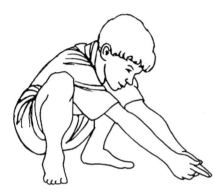

Praying Mantis Pose

"Who has seen a praying mantis? They have back legs that go up in a triangle shape, and large front pincers to hold what they are eating."

"If you squat down and let your knees open to the side, you have praying mantis back legs. To make the front pincers, clasp your hands as you lean forward and point them toward the floor. Stretch your arms forward. Take three deep breaths here."

Benefits: Praying Mantis Pose opens the hips and shoulders. It also develops balance.

2.   Dead Bug Pose

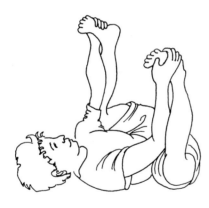

Dead Bug Pose

"If you keep your eyes open as you walk around outside, you might spot a dead bug. Of course, it might not really be dead—insects have their bones on the outside of their bodies (exoskeletons) and they do not grow. So they have to climb out of when they grow too big for them!"

"Lie on your back, bend your knees, and grab your feet with your hands. Gently pull your feet toward your chest. Take two deep breaths here. Now straighten out your legs so we can do this again."

Benefits: Dead Bug Pose opens the hips and stretches the inner thigh muscles. It also shows kids how silly yoga can be!

3.   Crow Pose (*Kakasana*)

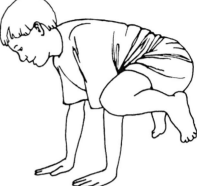

"The crow is an intelligent, strong bird with large wings. Let's see how you can use your abdominal muscles to be a crow."

"Squat down with your feet under your hips. Lean forward and tuck the top part of your arms between your legs. Now press your arms out and your knees in. Can you feel how strong this makes you? Now slowly lean forward on your hands. Come up to your tiptoes, perhaps you would like to life one leg off the floor. Don't lift your hips too high or you will be a diving bird! Your legs are balancing on your bent arms—which is why this pose is called an arm balance. If your body wants to try, lift both feet off the mat while balancing on your arms. Slowly come down and try it again. Often a pose is easier to do the second time around."

Crow Pose

Note: Students may want to try to jump back into Plank Pose from Crow Pose.

Benefits: Crow Pose builds abdominal (core) and arm strength. It also develops balance, focus, and self-confidence.

4.   Eagle (*Garudasana*)

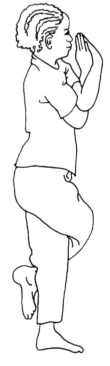

"*Garuda*, which is Sanskrit and translated as 'eagle', was a mythical bird of the gods. Let's see if we can wrap ourselves up with energy and feel strong like an eagle. What is our national bird? Do you know what bird Benjamin Franklin thought should be our national bird? (The wild turkey)"

"Being an eagle is not easy, so we will do this pose in two parts. Stand in Mountain Pose. Breathe your arms out to your side and move them out in front of you. First we need wings. Wrap your right arm over your left arm and clasp hands. Now bend your elbows and draw your clasped hands toward your face. Can you raise your hands in front of your face like a sharp eagle bill? If you like, you can now raise your left foot and lean it against your right leg. Now when you have your balance, think of yourself balancing high on a cliff and wrap your left foot around your standing leg. Now you are an eagle!"

Eagle Pose

Benefits: Eagle Pose improves balance and concentration. It also strengthens the legs and stretches the shoulders and upper back muscles.

5.   Wolf Pose

"Sometimes it is fun to use what we know about yoga to come up with our own poses. Wolf Pose is a pose created by a fifth grader. When you think of a wolf, what comes into your mind? She thought of him howling in the wilderness."

"Sit back on your feet with your arms, like front legs of a wolf, stretching down to the earth. Arch your head back and feel the stretch in the front of your body and throat. Now howl to the moon. After a good howl, take a deep breath and stretch toward the sky once more."

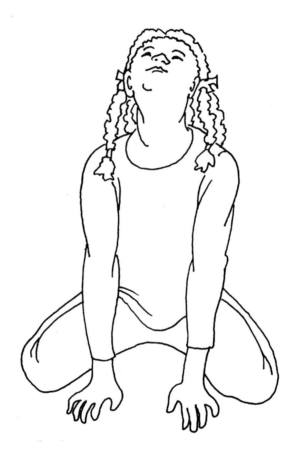

Wolf Pose

Note: Invite the kids to make up a pose for next week and do one or two at the end of the practice.

Benefits: Wolf Pose stretches the shoulders and front of the body. It also invites people to bring their creativity to the practice.

J.   Theme 10: Poses that Kick

Kids love to kick and jump and run. This theme works to draw their attention to the opportunities for kicking in yoga. It is probably not what they expect, which holds their interest as they wait for what they imagine the kick will be.

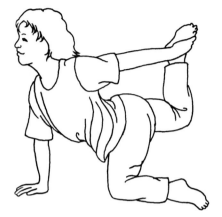

Suggestions for What to Say

1.   Spinal Twist Kick

"Come to your hands and knees, with your back flat just like a table. How could we kick from here?"

Spinal Twist Kick

"As you breathe in, reach your right arm out in front. As you breathe out, kick out your left leg. Now, reach your right arm over your back, bend your left leg so the foot is pointing up, and grab your left foot. Can you kick your left foot into your right hand? Breathe. Now slowly lower your arm and leg, come back to a flat back and then do a cat stretch. Come back to a flat back and let's kick with the other side."

Benefits: This pose is a gentle spinal twist. It also provides an opportunity to practice balance and concentration.

2.   Side Kick

"How could we turn that kick on its side? Roll over onto your bent right leg and straighten your left leg. Use your right arm to hold you up. As you take *your* next breath in, bend your left leg back so you can reach around and grab your left foot with your left hand. Kick into your hand as you raise your leg off the mat. Now come down so we can try that one more time. Now roll back to your hands and knees to a flat back, and try the other side."

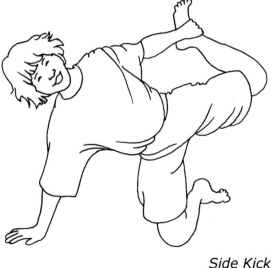

Benefits: This pose stretches the leg and shoulder muscles. It also builds balance and coordination.

Side Kick

3.   King Dancer (*Natarajasana*)

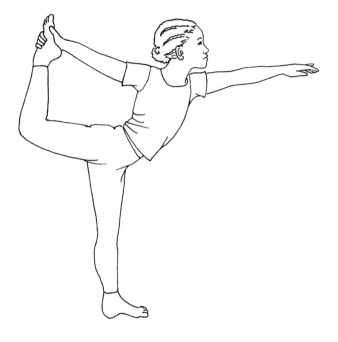

King Dancer

"Dancers can move and jump quickly so they need good balance. Let's practice a kick while balancing on one foot, just like a dancer might do. How do you think that might look?"

"To do King Dancer Pose, or perhaps you would like to do Queen Dancer Pose, bend your left leg back and reach around with your left hand and grab your ankle or the top of your foot. Breathe in and raise your right hand out in front of you for balance. As you breathe out, slowly bend forward from the waist and lift your back leg. Take several deep breaths. Now let's kick on the other side."

Note: This pose can be done with one hand resting on a friend's shoulder or a wall.

Benefits: King Dancer Pose helps develop focus, balance, and concentration. It also stretches the legs and abdomen.

4.   Bow Pose (*Dhanurasana*)

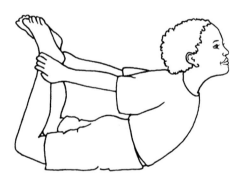

Bow Pose

"If you lie on your stomach, how could you make your body look like an archer's bow?"

"Bend your knees and reach back to grab your ankles or the top of your feet. When you breathe out, kick your feet into your hands and lift your chest off the floor. Can you kick a little more and lift your legs a little higher? Now you are like the bow—stretched and ready to release an arrow. Next time you breathe out, lower down to your mat and rest for two breaths. Let's try it again."

Benefits: Bow Pose in an energizing pose that opens the chest and increases flexibility of the spine and back. It also stretches the muscles in the legs and abdomen.

5.   Swimmer 2 Pose

"An important part of swimming is using your legs to kick. Imagine that you are in a beautiful lake surrounded by pine trees. Feel the sun warming your body as you take a breath in, and stretch your right arm and hold it there. Now as you breathe out, raise your left leg. Reach around with your right hand and grab the top of your left foot or ankle. Kick into it like a swimmer kicking. Slowly release back to the floor."

"Now let's do the other side. Swimming is fun, so let's do this two more times. Let's imagine we are swimming in a calm ocean. Then we can imagine we are swimming in a wide, lazy river."

Benefits: The pose builds strength in the core and provides a spinal twist. It also exercises the imagination.

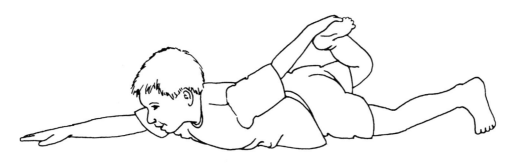

Swimmer 2

K.   Theme 11: Geometric Yoga

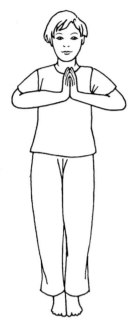

Kids have been studying shapes for year—it is one of the first ways they start to organize their world. Making shapes with the body is naturally interesting and fun to people.

Suggestions for What to Say:

1.   Straight Lines
a.   Mountain Pose (*Tadasana*)

"How can you make your body into one straight line?"
"Find a comfortable place for your feet and gently rock back and forth to find the point where you feel balanced and strong, like the base of a mountain. Roll your shoulders back, keep your eyes looking forward. How can you make the line longer? Breathe your hands up and reach for the clouds."

Benefits: Mountain Pose is a standing pose that helps with balance and good posture.

Mountain Pose

b.   Warrior 3 or "T" Pose

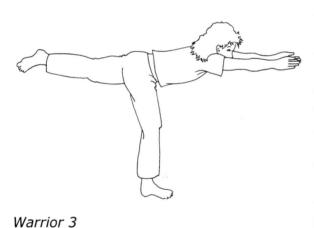

Warrior 3

"How can you move your body so that you make two straight lines?"
"Stand in Mountain Pose, with your arms reaching over your head. Shift all your weight into your right foot. Reach your left leg back so the toes point down on the mat. Take a deep inhale, and as you breathe out bend forward from the waist so that your arms go out like a 'T'. If your body would like, lift your back leg, so your whole body becomes the letter 'T'. Breathe your leg and arms down. Let's do it one more time."

Note: Kids can lean toward a friend and rest their arms on the friend's shoulders or a wall to feel the full stretch.

Benefits: Warrior 3 strengthens the legs and arms. It improves balance and builds stamina and confidence.

c.   Rocket 2 or Reverse Gate

"How might we make ourselves into a long line, but this time on an angle?"

"Stand on your knees. Now extend your right leg to the side and let your left palm drop to the floor. As you take a deep inhale, sweep your right arm over your head, next to your ear. If someone had a ruler, could they draw a line from the tip of your right hand to the heel of your right foot? Think of a rocket blasting out of your

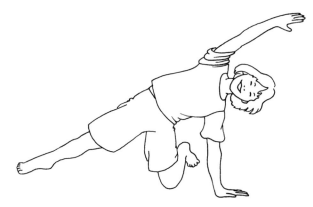

Rocket 2

right arm. Breathe in two long breaths. Sweep your arm down, and then let's do it once more. Now let's rest in Child's Pose for a few breaths. Come up to sitting when your body tells you it is time."

Benefits: Rocket Pose gives the body an intense side stretch. It also opens the chest.

2.   Triangles
a.   Downward Facing Dog (*Adho Mukha Svanasana*)

"How can you use your whole body to make one big triangle?"

"Get on your hands and knees with a flat back. Your hands are under your shoulders. Curl your toes under and push your hips up as your body forms one big triangle. Can you make the triangle a little taller by pushing your hips a little higher toward the sky? Let's be a big triangle in Down Dog for three breaths. Now lower your knees to the floor and sit back on your heels."

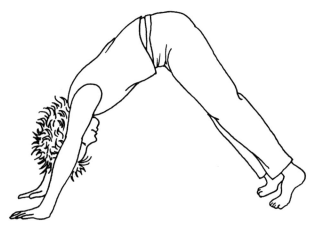

Down Dog

Benefits: Downward Facing Dog stretches from the hips down the backs of the legs. It also reverses the flow of blood so that the brain gets extra oxygen and nutrients.

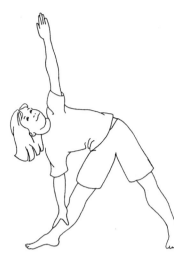

Triangle Pose

b.   Triangle Pose (*Trikonasana*)

"How can we use our bodies to be several triangles at once?"

"Stand facing the left side of the room with your feet wide apart. Turn your toes in like a duck and quack three times. Now turn the right foot so that it faces me at the front of the room. You may need to move your feet a little closer together to find a spot in which you feel balanced. As you take a deep inhale, sweep your left arm up then bend forward into Triangle Pose. You can rest your right hand on your thigh, or if it feels comfortable, find a place lower on your right leg. Count how many triangles you can see when I do it. Now face a partner and let's do it again. Count the triangles that your partner has made."

Benefits: Triangle Pose stretches the sides of the body and increases flexibility in the hips and spine.

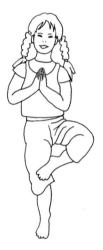

Tree Pose

c.   Tree Pose

"How can we make some triangles while we stand straight and tall?"

"Stand in Mountain Pose. Rock gently back and forth on your feet to find your balance point in the middle. How can we make a small triangle with one leg? We can do this pose in a number of ways. Choose what feels good for your body. Put all your weight on to your right foot. Find a *drishti* point, or a point at eye level that is not moving, to focus on. Now lift your left foot and rest it by your ankle, press it into your leg—either at your calf, above your knee, or high up on your thigh (not on your knee!) Think of your foot and your standing leg having a conversation—each one is active and pressing the other back. It makes a strong post on which you can stand. Now how can we make some triangles with our arms? Place your hands together in Prayer Pose at your chest and look down at your elbows! Slowly breathe your hands up, and keep your elbows bent. What shape do you see?"

Note: You can offer kids the challenge of doing this pose with their eyes closed, while looking at something that is moving, or while resting a hand on a friend's shoulder.

Benefits: Tree pose helps develop focus and concentration. It builds balance and leg strength.

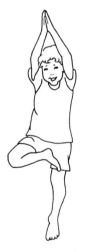

Tree Pose

2.   Circles and Arcs
a.   Snowball Pose

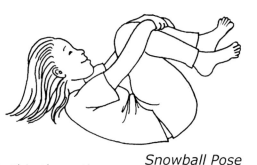

"Would you like to make silly circles that move? Let's make snowballs."

"Lie on your back, pull your knees into your chest, and wrap your arms around your legs. Pull your head up so your body is in a tight ball. Now you can either rock from side to side, or you can rock with more energy so that your body moves around in a circle. We are going to do this three times in each direction. See how big you can make your snowball!"

Snowball Pose

Benefits: Snowball Pose gently releases the muscles in the lower back and massages the internal organs.

b.   Bridge (*Setu Bandha*)

"Now lie flat on your mat. How can you make your body into a semi, or half, circle? Let's make a bridge."

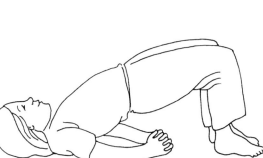

"Pull your feet in so they are directly under your knees. Your toes should be pointed forward. Roll your shoulders back, so that there is a space under your neck (this protects the bones in your neck, the cervical vertebrae). We have seven cervical vertebrae—guess how many a giraffe has? It also has 7! Now press your arms into the floor and lift your hips off the floor, like a bridge. You can push your hands up under your back and be a suspension bridge, too. Take two full breaths here, and then roll down to the mat, as if your vertebrae (the bones in your spine) were a string of pearls, resting one pearl at a time on the mat. Let's make another bridge, this time clasping our hands under our backs on the mat."

Bridge Pose

Note: There are students who may be comfortable doing a full backbend at this point. Backbend is an advanced pose and should not be done without proper supervision.

Benefits: Bridge Pose is an energizing pose. It also stretches the abdominal muscles and strengthens the muscles in the back. It stretches the muscles in the legs too, which make it a good pose to do after sitting at a desk all day.

c.   Arches Pose

"An arch is another kind of half circle. What sort of arches do we see outside? To make a big arch, find a partner."

"Each of you stands on your knees at the end of a mat, and you are both facing the same direction. You are far enough apart so you can reach out and touch hands. Now each person extends the outside leg straight out to the side. Each of you sweeps your outside arm up and over your head so you can clasp your friend's hand. You have made an arch, or another half circle. Now practice breathing in the same rhythm as your partner. After three breaths together, release and switch places on the mat. Now make another arch."

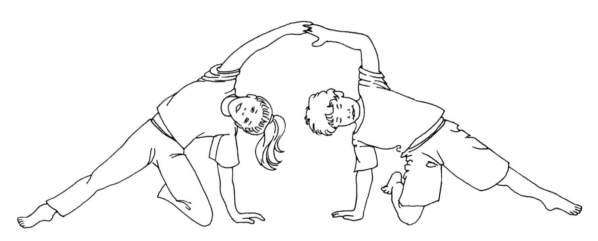

Arches Pose

Note: You can also do this pose standing.

Benefits: This pose provides a side stretch and opens the chest. It also builds cooperation and brings attention to the breath.

L.   Theme 12: Out of This World Yoga

The idea of being able to leave the planet or thinking about what is out in space intrigues people of all ages—especially kids. Grouping poses together that help people think about somewhere beyond our planet is a real crowd pleaser. It stretches their bodies and their imaginations!

Suggestions of What to Say:

1.   Crescent Moon

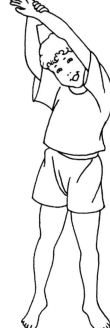

"Does anyone know what phase the moon is in now? Maybe you can look outside tonight and see. What does a crescent moon look like?"

"Let's start in Mountain Pose, with our arms down at our sides. As you slowly take a breath in, raise your arms toward the moon, stretching from your feet to the tips of your fingers. Imagine someone leaning down from a cloud and gently pulling you up. Take another breath in and put your hands together, with the index finger pointing up and the fingers interlaced. As you breathe out, bend toward your right side and make a crescent moon. Breathe back to center as you stretch toward the sky. Then slowly bend to the other side. Let's do that again."

Crescent Moon

Benefits: Crescent Moon Pose is an energizing pose. It stretches the sides of your body (a lateral stretch) and the spine. It also builds strength in the abdominal area (core).

2.   Star Pose (*Utthita Tadasana*)

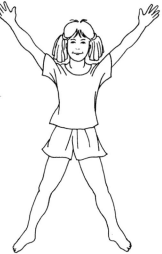

"What makes a star shine in the night sky? Who knows the name of the star closest to earth? (The sun) Let's make ourselves into stars giving off a lot of energy."

"Stand and spread your feet apart. Press your feet into the earth. Let's raise our arms and reach out, as if someone is gently pulling our arms into space. Raise your head tall. Take a deep breath in and feel the energy moving from your arms and legs. Slowly release the breath. Let's do this three times and see how brightly we can glow."

Benefits: This pose energizes the body and provides a good stretch for the legs, shoulders, and arms. It also opens the chest, which allows for deeper breathing.

Star Pose

3.   Rocket 2

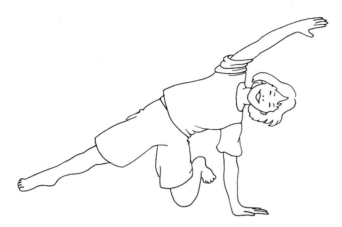

Rocket 2

"If you wanted to leave the planet, how would you do it? Let's get our bodies set up for Rocket Pose and see how far we can blast."

"Stand on your knees. Extend your right leg out to your side and allow you left palm to rest on the floor by your side. Now take a deep breath in and sweep your right arm over your head, next to your ear. If someone had a ruler, could she draw a line from the tip of your right hand to your right foot? Take two long breaths. Come down out of the pose, and then let's blast off once more on the same side. Now let's rest in Child's Pose for a few breaths. Come up to sitting when your body tells you it is time. Now let's see if the other side blasts us to a different galaxy!"

Benefits: Rocket 2 gives the body an intense side stretch. It also opens your chest.

4.   Sun Salute (*Surya Namaskar*)

"Now we are going to do a series of flowing poses and are called a 'Sun Salute'. It is a wonderful way to awaken the spirit and the energy of a new day."

a.   Mountain Pose (*Tadasana*)

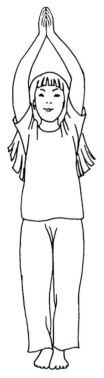

Mountain Pose

"Mountains are built of rocks that have been pushed out of the earth. Do mountains sway in the breeze like trees? Do they move around like water? We are going to stand like a tall, strong mountain"

"Find a comfortable place for your feet and gently rock back and forth to find the point where you feel balanced and strong, the base of a mountain. Roll your shoulders back so your chest has a lot of room for air to fill your lungs when you breathe. Now breathe your hands up and reach for the clouds.

b.   Forward Bend (*Uttanasana*)

"Bend your knees so they are soft. Now as you breathe out, melt your arms down so that your fingers are touching the mat. Bend your knees a little more so that your palms rest on the mat."

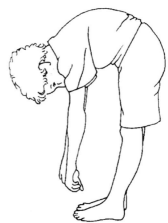

c.   Lunge

"Now with hands are on either side of your left foot, step your right foot back."

Forward Bend

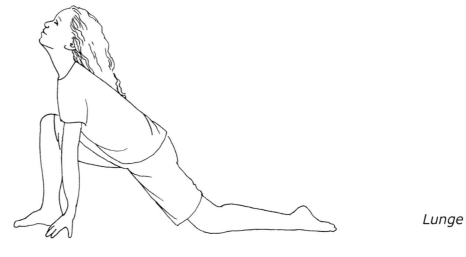

Lunge

d.   Plank Pose

"Now, step your left leg back to meet your right. You are now in Plank Pose. There should be a straight line from your head, across your back, and down your legs. Take a deep breath and see if you can feel it move in that straight line down your body."

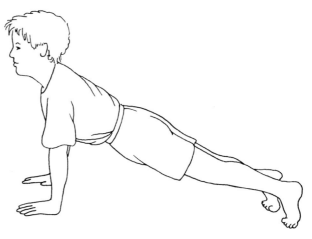

Plank Pose

93

e.   Upward Facing Dog (*Urdhva Mukha Svanasana*)

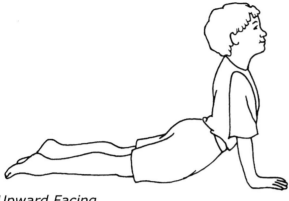

"Lower yourself to the mat, and then use your arms to lift your chest and hips off the ground. Breathe!"

Upward Facing Dog

f.   Down Dog

"Now curl your toes under and push back into Down Dog. Your hands are right under your shoulders. Push your hips up high to the sky. Stretch your heels down toward the mat. Let's stay here for 3 full breaths, breathing in and then out is one breath."

Down Dog

g.   To complete:

"Now walk or hop both feet up between your hands, so you are back in Forward Bend. Slowly roll up to Mountain Pose. Extend your hands over your head, and then lower them to your chest in a folded prayer position (*Angali Mudra*)."

Note: Repeat as you like—Yael finds that kids enjoy one or two flows. Some yogis do 108 to start the day!

Benefits: Doing the Sun Salutation series allows you to stretch and to strengthen many muscles in the body. Repeating the sequence can create an energizing group of postures as the kids become familiar with the flow.

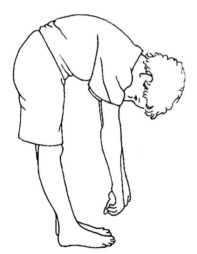

Forward Bend

IV.   Relaxation

It is very important to leave at least ten minutes at the end of a practice for relaxation. Kids, just like adults, need to give their nervous systems an opportunity to calm down and to absorb the benefits of yoga. The relaxation section offers everyone an opportunity to learn how to relax by themselves.

Suggestions for What to Say:

A.   Sequence 1

1.   Seated Twist

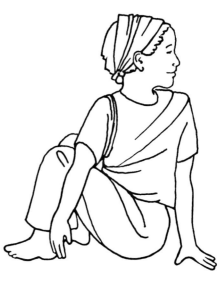

"Now we are at the relaxing part of our practice. The next poses are good to do before you go to bed, if you feel like you are getting sick, or if you need to relax."

"Let's sit with our legs out in front with a straight spine. Now bend your knees and put your feet flat on the mat (or the knees can be down to one side). Place both hands on the floor to your left and take a deep breath. As you release the breath, slowly look over your left shoulder. Now you are squeezing the blood out of your stomach, kidneys, and liver with the twist. Take another breath. Release back to center. As you untwist, fresh blood is going to your organs! Twists are healthy for your organs."

Seated Twist

"If your knees are down to one side, pretend a crane is over you lifting your knees over to the other side. Then twist to the right and look over your right shoulder."

Benefits: Twists stimulate the internal organs. As you untwist, the organs are infused with blood filled with oxygen and nutrients. Twists also strengthen the spine.

2.   Seated Forward Bend (*Janu Sirsansana*)

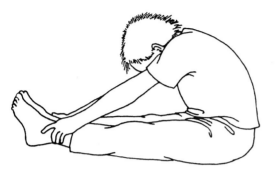

Seated Forward Bend

"After you twist something, it is a good idea to straighten it out again. How could we make our spine long and straight while we are still sitting?"

"Straighten your legs in front of you and shake them out. Now pull your right foot up and rest it next to your left thigh. Put your hands on your hips and start to melt forward over your straight leg. It may feel better to lift your left knee up a few inches as you do. Listen to your body and your muscles so you know when to stop bending. Take a deep breath and feel your spine get longer! As you exhale, melt a little more. Now let's do the other side."

Benefits: Forward bends are very calming. They also stretch the spine and hamstrings.

3.   Final Relaxation (*Savasana*)

Note: It is important to give people enough time to really relax. We have found that everyone enjoys this part—they appreciate the quiet and the space just to "be". Everyone will enjoy it if you allow a full ten minutes for *Savasana*.

"Are you ready to try a pose many adults find really hard to do? I think you can do it though, because you are all good yogis. We do Final Relaxation, or *Savasana*, to allow our bodies to absorb all the benefits of our yoga practice. You may like to think of your body as a sponge, as Lilias Folan suggests, as we lie quietly and let our muscles relax. (1) We allow our minds to find calmness. I am going to give you some ideas of things to think about to allow your mind to be calm."

a.   Tensing/Relaxing Exercise

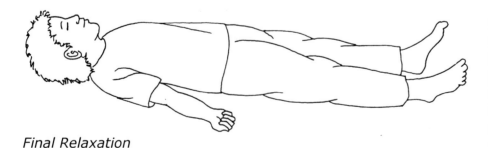

Final Relaxation

"Let's lie down with our arms out to ours sides, palms facing up. Our feet fall open to the side. Allow your eyes to close.

On your next breath in, tense the muscles in your hands as tightly as you can. Now as you breathe out, let them relax. On your *next* breath in, tense the muscles in both your hands and feet. As you breathe out, let everything relax. And on your next inhale, tense every muscle in your body—even the 80 muscles in your face—as tightly as you can! And as you breathe out, relax everything.

Now we are ready for *Savasana*."

b.   Rainbow Relaxation

Note: You may want to read this aloud to the kids.

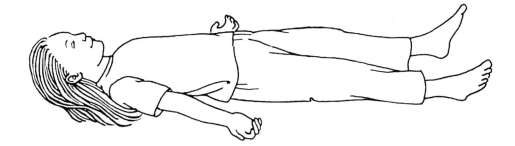

Final Relaxation

"Imagine your name written across the sky in all the colors of the rainbow. Slowly your name gets bigger. Watch the red, the orange, the yellow, the green, the blue, the indigo, and the violet of the rainbow glistening through the raindrops. Each color may hold a different healing energy—you don't have to know for sure what they are, but they may include loving, caring, forgiving sharing, hoping, protecting, soothing, or maybe something else you don't even think of! Slowly, the glistening rainbow of your name comes toward you, covering you like a cool (or warm, depending on the season!) blanket. The colors melt into you, filling your cells with the healing, rainbow energy. As you lie in this final relaxing pose, all these healing energies will spread to all the cells in your body. So use this quiet time to allow this to happen. In a few minutes, I will tell you when we are done."

After ten minutes say, "Now slowly start to wiggle your fingers and toes. Stretch your hands over your head and stretch from tip to toe. Now roll over on to your side and take several deep breaths here. When you are ready, help yourself up to sitting and sit in Easy Pose. The last part of a yoga practice is to place your hands together in *Angali Mudra* and bow to each other. Together we say, 'Namaste', which means, 'The goodness in me bows to, or acknowledges, the goodness in you.' We all have goodness in us, and it is nice when someone else sees it!

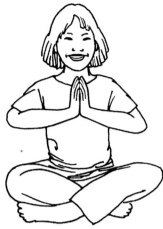

"You can remember some of these relaxation poses if you want to calm yourself or just find a settling feeling."

Benefits: Savasana is a key part of any yoga practice. It allows the body to absorb and to integrate the many benefits of yoga. It allows everyone the time to practice a quiet time and feel the effects. Visualization exercises can help guide the kids through the process.

Easy Pose in Angali Mudra

B.   Sequence 2

1.   Circle of Knees to Circle of Arms

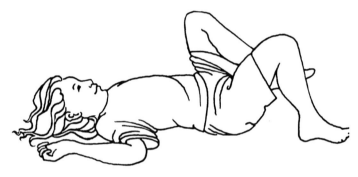

"Now we are at the relaxing part of our practice. The next poses are also good to do before you go to bed, if you feel that you are getting sick, or if you need to relax."

"Let's lie down on our backs and stretch out. Draw your right foot in so that it rests right under your right knee. Pretend there is a crayon of your

Circle of Knees

favorite color (or a spring/fall/holiday color) on your knee. Let's draw big circles on the ceiling. Draw three circles in one direction and three circles in the other. Now, straighten the leg and let's do the other side with a different color."

"Now choose a festive color and pretend that crayon is on your right elbow. Raise your arms and draw three big circles on the wall. Now draw the circles in the other direction. Now use the other elbow to color."

Note: You can extend this activity by imagining crayons on the toes, fingers, and shoulders. You can also circle both knees together.

Benefits: This pose lubricates the joints in the hips, knees, and arms. It is also a fun way to introduce visualization exercises.

2.   Knees into Chest

"Let's make our backs smile. From a lying down position, how can we make our backs into a smile shape?"

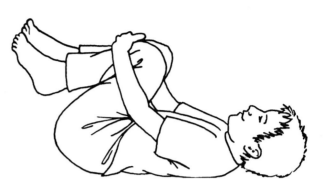

Knees to Chest

"Pull your knees into your chest and wrap your arms around them in a big hug. To make an even bigger smile for your back, raise your head while you hug your knees. Take a big breath in and then slowly release it! This releases the muscles in your back. On your next exhale, stretch out on your mat. Then let your back smile one more time."

Benefits: This pose also lubricates the joints in the hips, knees, and arms, while engaging the participation of the visual imagination.

1.   Final Relaxation (*Savasana*)

Note: It's important to give everyone enough time to really relax. You will discover how much people enjoy the quiet time and space you are offering them. We encourage you to allow at least 10 minutes for *Savasana.*

a.   Eye Warming

"Let's do a relaxation pose that allows our bodies to absorb all the benefits of our yoga practice—just like a sponge. We lie down and allow ourselves to be peacefully still as we let our muscles relax. We let our minds grow calm. I am going to give you some ideas that can help calm your mind."

"Let's lie down with our feet out to the side. Rub your palms together until you feel some heat. When your palms are really warm, cup them over your eyes for a minute. Let the heat relax your eyes. Then let your arms rest on the floor, palms open.

Eye Warming

b.   Relax Your Feet Visualization

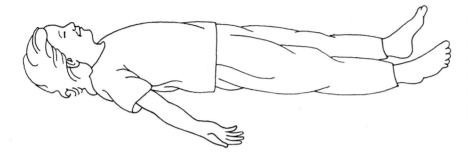

"Listen as I help you to relax the rest of you." (Say this slowly so people have time to relax each part.)

Final Relaxation

"Wiggle your toes, then let them doze,
Relax feet to this gentle beat,
Relax your heels, like sunning seals
Relax your legs like mama birds sitting on eggs
Relax your knees, just say please
Relax your hips, don't do flips
Relax your bones, with gentle tones
Relax your muscles, from their tussles
Relax your nerves, with healing herbs
Relax your tummy, just say yummy
Relax your heart, it's a good start
Relax your ribs, like babies' bibs
Relax your chest, let it rest
Relax your back, like a cuddle sack
Relax your back, your neck and spine
Relax your spine like a tall limber pine
Relax your trapezius 'cuz it's the easiest
Relax your shoulder before you get older
Relax your arms with wizards' charms
Relax your elbow, let it swing low
Relax your hand without a demand
Relax your finger, yet it linger
Relax your palm, like a gentle psalm
Relax your jaw let it thaw
Relax your nose let it doze
Relax your skin, tuck it in
Relax your chin, just as your skin
Relax your mind, in front and behind
Relax your face like silk and lace
Relax your eyes, like warm summer skies
Relax your ears with joyful tears
Relax your brain like a gentle spring rain"

"After a few minutes say, "Now slowly start to wiggle your fingers and toes. Stretch your hands over your head and stretch from tip to toe. Then roll over on to your side and take several deep breaths here. When you are ready, help yourself up to sitting and sit in Easy Pose. The last part of a yoga practice is to place your hands together in *Angali Mudra* and bow to each other. Together we say, '*Namaste*', which means, 'The goodness in me bows to, or acknowledges, the goodness in you.' We all have goodness in us, and it is nice when someone else notices it!"

"When you need to help yourself calm down, these are some poses you can do to let a feeling of relaxation come to you."

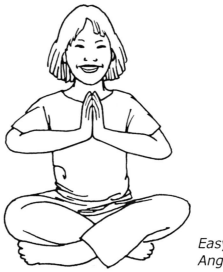

Easy Pose in Angali Mudra

Benefits: Final Relaxation allows kids to just let go—they learn that they can create a calmness within themselves. Doing Final Relaxation with some guided activity in the beginning invites kids to become a part of the process.

C.   Sequence 3

1.   Lying Down Twist

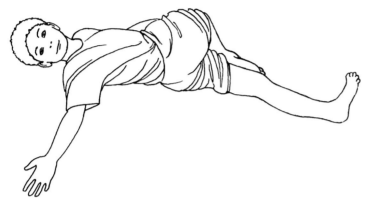

"Before we end a practice, we should clean things up. So let's help clean our abdominal organs by squeezing them out and letting new blood flow back in, just like squeezing out a sponge."

"Stretch out on your mat. Put your right foot on top of your left thigh. Take your left hand and gently pull your right leg over to the left side. Look over your right arm. Take a few breaths here as your organs are squeezed a little like a sponge. Now straighten your right leg and shake it out. Take a deep breath as new blood flows into your kidneys, liver, and stomach. Now let's squeeze the other side."

Lying Down Twist

Benefits: Twists are calming and stimulate the internal organs. They also stretch the intercostal (side) muscles between the ribs, which allows for deeper breathing.

2.   Easy Bridge Pose

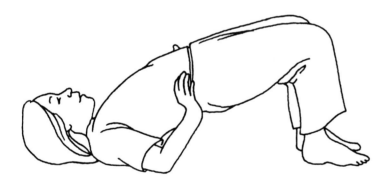

"After doing a twist, it is good to get our spines straight again. Put your feet under your knees and gently lift your hips toward the sky. Your arms are on the floor helping to push your back up. Take two breaths here. Think of the bones in your spine, your vertebrae, as beads on a necklace. Starting with your neck vertebrae, slowly roll them down to the floor, one bead at a time. Allow you legs to straighten."

Easy Bridge Pose

Benefits: Doing an Easy Bridge Pose after a twist allows the spine to straighten and lengthen. You want to go into Final Relaxation with a straight spine.

3.   Final Relaxation (*Savasana*)

Note: It is important to give everyone enough time to really relax. Take the time to discover how much people appreciate the permission to enjoy the quiet. We encourage you to allow a full ten minutes to enjoy the final relaxation part of the practice.

a.   Shells

"I am going to give each of you two shells (or pebbles) to hold in your palms. Take a moment and explore how each one feels in your hands. Yoga is about being aware of what is going on with your body, so as we relax in *Savasana*, you can think about how the shell feels resting on your palm."

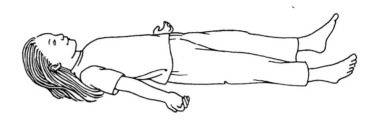

Final Relaxation

"The more you practice the next pose, the better you become at doing it. Did you know for some adults it is very hard to lie still? But you are all good yogis, so I think we can give our bodies this special time to absorb all the benefits of our yoga practice."

"Let's lie down with our feet out to the side. Your hands are at your sides, with a shell resting in each palm. While we do Savasana, let your hands be open and not moving. I am going to give you some ideas of things to think about as we relax."

b.   Yoga Smile Visualization

"Let your jaw relax. Let your tongue float in your mouth. Have a sense that the back of your mouth is hollow—full of good energy. Let this good, "smiling" energy move from the back of your mouth down into your throat, chest, mid section, and stomach. Let this good, warm, smiling energy tingle and mingle into your inner organs and find its way into hidden places that need a little of your inner sunshine." (Pause.)

"Let your muscles...relax...more fully, and let the inner
        warmth melt away any extra tension you might have.
Let yourself relax more deeply, more sweetly, more com-
        pletely. Let yourself be soft like wax.
Relax your toes, wiggle 'em, and let 'em doze.
Relax your feet with restful heat.
Relax your legs like hens hatch eggs.
Relax your stomach, thin and thick.
Relax your torso, don't force so.
Relax your arms like night on farms.
Relax your head, put it to bed."

D.   More Visualization Exercises for Savasana

1.   Deep Relaxation

Edward Hall, in his book *The Dance of Life*, describes the Japanese concept of "MA" as pauses, or silences that carry meaning and are significant. During "quiet time," stuff is happening. The body is processing. Leave spaces during yoga. It is not a race.

Here is a relaxation/visualization sequence that allows you to practice the art of meaningful pausing.

"Some say that twenty minutes of deep relaxation can be as helpful as two hours of sleep. Even a minute of calm relaxation can offer you unexpected energy later in the day!"

> "Lie back in Final Relaxation position. Gently tense your left foot. Relax it.
> (Pause.)
> Let any extra tension run out your foot, down your toes, and out of your body.
> (Pause.)
> Gently tense your right foot.
> (Pause.)
> Relax it.
> (Pause.)
> Let any extra tension run out your foot, down your toes, and out of your body.
> (Pause.)
> Gently tense both feet. Let them relax as any extra tension runs out your feet, down your toes, and out of your body.
> (Pause.)
> Gently tense your left calf, then your right calf. Release them.
> (Pause.)
> Let any extra tension run out of your calves, out of your feet, down your toes, and out of your body.
> (Pause.)
> Continue this with the knees, thighs, buttocks, stomach, and chest.
> "Now, gently tense your shoulders, then your arms, wrists, hands, and fingers."
> (Pause.)
> Pretend, in a playful, 'make-believe way,' that you are holding in this tension some left-over anger, anxiety, fear, or some other unsettling thing that you no longer need, if you ever did.
> (Pause.)

Gently make them a little even MORE tense!
(Pause.)
And now, let all that tension go! Relax and release your shoulders, your arms, wrists, hands, and fingers, and let that tension just run out your fingers."
(Pause.)

"Now, tense your whole back, your spine, your neck, your face—make a tight, mean face! Really scrunch it up! Oh, that face is tense! Wow! And now, let it go. Relax! And let that tension run down your spine, gentling it and soothing it, and let it run out your toes and fingers, out of your body, out of your life, to wherever it is good for it to go. And rest. You've earned it."

2.   Floating and Sinking

"OK, now, just let your body float. You are floating on a cloud. You are floating on a magic cloud, gently and safely holding you up, and all cares are leaving you. The cloud is taking you to a place of comfort, but don't worry about where right now. Just enjoy floating...resting... and you are now gently resting on the earth. Gently sinking into the soft, safe, earth. You can pretend you are getting heavier and heavier, more and more relaxed, sinking down into a deep, calm, restful place. Let your body restore itself, and rest, and relax."
(Pause.)

After many gentle breaths have passed, say, "Now slowly start to wiggle your fingers and toes. Stretch your hands over your head and stretch from tip to toe. Now roll over on to your side and take several deep breaths here. When you are ready, help yourself up to sitting and sit in Easy Pose. The last part of a yoga practice is to place your hands together in *Angali Mudra* and bow to each other. Together we say, '*Namaste*', which means, 'The goodness in me bows to, or acknowledges, the goodness in you.' We all have goodness in us, and it is a good feeling when you acknowledge it in someone else!"

"You can remember some of these relaxation poses if you want to calm yourself or just find a settling feeling."

Benefits: *Savasana* is a key part of a yoga practice. It allows the body to absorb and to integrate the many benefits of yoga. It allows the kids to practice a quiet time and feel the effects. Visualization exercises can help guide everyone through the process.

V. More Yoga Fun

The following yoga exercises can be woven into any practice. Variety allows you to adapt to different situations and to keep the practice fresh.

Suggestions for What To Say:

A. Yoga at the Wall

Wall poses give us a chance to move off the mats. We do the easier wall poses as a larger group. Only attempt the more difficult poses, like handstand or headstand, if you have an adult to supervise a smaller group of students.

1. Half Forward Bend (*Ardha Uttanasana*)

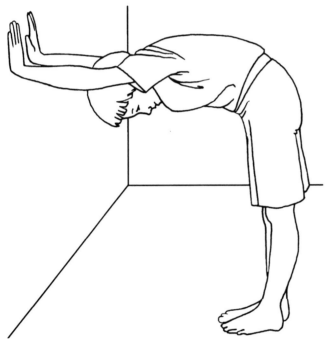

"Doing yoga poses at the wall is fun, and it also strengthens muscles to keep your body from getting hurt."

"Find a spot at the wall you would like to touch with your palms. Stand about three feet from the wall and slowly bend halfway down, so that you can feel the wall on the palms of your hand. Did you know that your spine actually goes up into your head to the point where your nose is? So as you bend over, don't drop your head and don't lift it—just let it be a continuation of your spine. Push into the wall with your palms and into the floor with your feet. Take three deep breaths here."

Half Forward Bend

Benefits: This pose lengthens the spine and stretches the muscles in the arms, the legs, and the back. It also is a beginning step toward building confidence in balance poses.

2.   Reverse Handstand

"Close your eyes and imagine in your mind what this pose would look like if you turned it upside down. You are going to get to see the world from a different perspective—this may be a good pose to do when you want to solve a problem in a new way!"

"Open your eyes and sit against the wall with your legs out on the floor. Notice in your mind where your heels are. Slowly move forward onto your knees and put your palms flat on the floor in that spot. Now begin to walk up the wall, so that you are standing on your hands. See how far you can walk up the wall, and then walk down so that your body looks like the corner of a box. The pose you are now doing is the opposite of the last one! Come down and try it again."

Note: Some students may feel comfortable going into a handstand in which they are facing away from the wall. An adult should supervise such advanced poses.

Benefits: A major benefit of this inversion pose is that it reverses the blood flow in the body. It sends extra blood to the brain and moves the lymph around the body, which helps fight infections. It builds strength in the arms and wrist, while building confidence.

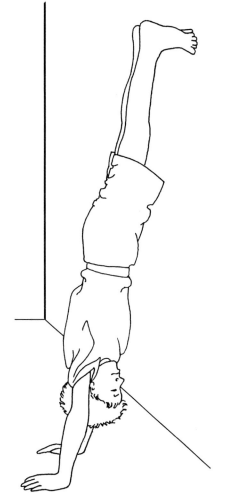

Reverse Handstand

3.   Half Moon (*Ardha Chandrasana*)

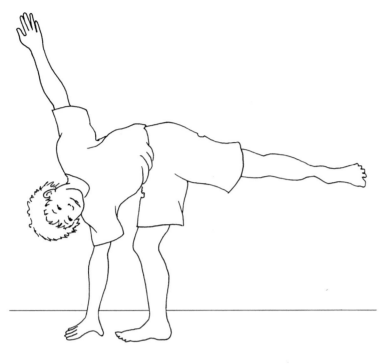

Half Moon

"Does anyone know what phase the moon is in right now? Remember to look outside tonight or first thing tomorrow morning. We are going to be open like a bright moon, letting our energy shine out."

"There are two ways to do **this** pose. Stand close to a **wall** with more than enough room to spread your arms. Lean against the wall with your feet out like a duck (you may want to quack three times). Now turn your right foot so that it points to the right and is lined up with the wall. Raise your arms to shoulder level. Look at your right foot—now make a commitment not to move it. That foot is your stable base for rising into a shining moon! Slowly tilt over toward the right, using the wall to keep your back straight. Reach down as far as you can with your right hand. Keep both hips against the wall and feel the energy shine out. Take two breaths here, come back up, and do the other side."

"The other way to be a moon is to stand an arm's length away from the wall. Bend half-way down so that your right palm is flat on the wall. Lift your left leg so that it is parallel to the floor. Now slowly breathe your left hand up so that it points toward the ceiling. As you do this your left hip will slowly turn up so it faces the wall in front of you. After two breaths, lower your right arm and leg, and do the other side."

Benefits: Half Moon Pose builds strength in the legs. It also develops a sense of balance and concentration. It opens the chest while building a sense of power and confidence.

4.   Legs up the Wall (*Virpareti Karani*)

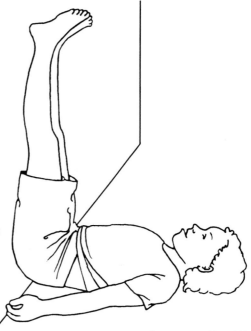

"After doing poses that build heat and energize your body, it is important to pause and let your body absorb the benefits of what you have done. How could we pause at the wall?"

"Let's sit about five inches from the wall. Slowly release your back down by resting on your elbows, while you swing your legs up the wall. You may want to close your eyes as you breathe for about 10 breaths. Then let your legs drop out to the side. Take some breaths here. When you are ready, pull your knees in toward you so that your feet are resting on the wall. Then roll over to your side where you started."

Benefits: Lifting your legs above your head increases blood flow to the brain. This pose is restorative and calming to the nervous system and the mind.

Legs up the Wall

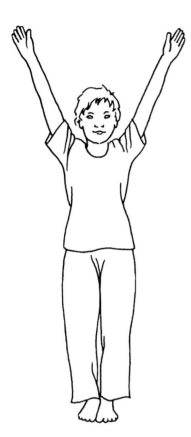

B. Yoga Games

1.   Alphabet Game

"Close your eyes and picture the first letter or your name. Now open your eyes and try to make your body into that letter. You may use your middle or last name if that seems more fun."

"What letters could two people make? Find a partner and make a capital A. What other letters can we make?"

"Now let's see if we can spell out the words "YOGA IS FUN!" using people for letters."

Note: It is possible to spell out "Yoga is Fun!" with a little bit of experimenting and a lot of laughter. You may want to bring a camera to photograph the wonderful letters.

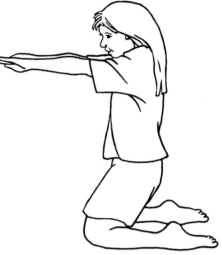

Letter "Z"

Letter "Y"

2.   Chain Game

"We are going to link ourselves together in a chain. We will make lines of about six people and get on our hands and knees. Leave enough space between you so that when you stretch your right arm out you can rest your hand on the hip of the person in front of you. Now carefully stretch out your left leg and put it over the shoulder of the person in back of you. Now everyone is connected. Can we make the chain move by all breathing in together and then exhaling together?"

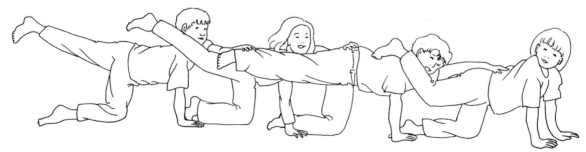

Chain Game

3. Awareness Games

"*Awareness* is the key!"
—Lilias Folan

Here are three simple exercises to lay the groundwork for increasing self-awareness that can follow naturally during yoga practice. These can be practiced while lying in Final Relaxation Pose or sitting in Easy Pose. This sequence will allow children to deepen their discovery of the great yoga experience of becoming more rested and alert at the same time.

a.   Noticing Game 1

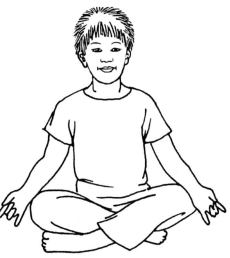

"Close your eyes and notice your body. You don't have to change it, or stop it from changing. Simply notice it. And begin to notice, more and more, your breathing. You don't have to make yourself breathe correctly, or stop yourself from breathing more easily...simply notice your breath going in, and going out...and are there any tense places in your body that you notice? You don't have to do anything to release them, or stop yourself from releasing them, simply notice your breathing, and your stomach, going up and down."
(Two breaths.)

Easy Pose

"And notice your chest, the breath going in and out, and in there, your heart is beating, just beautifully, patiently, wonderfully. You don't have to make it do something, or stop it from doing something —just notice how it knows how to beat, all on its own."
(Two breaths.)

"And clearly notice your head, and there it is—you don't have to fix it, or stop yourself from fixing it—right now, just let it rest comfortably."
(Two breaths.)

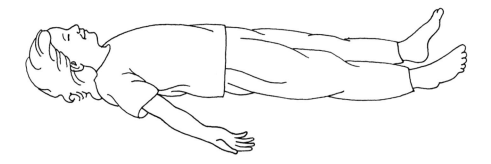

Final Relaxation

b.   Noticing Game 2

"And now, notice your feelings—whatever they are. They can be easy, or uncomfortable, or surprising, or mixed up—you don't have to try to change them or fix them right now, or make them be a certain way. Just accept them. If they change, they can change—simply notice them, and notice your breathing, your stomach, your body, your feelings."
(Two or three breaths.)

"And notice if there are things in life you want. You might want to be safe, and warm, and comfortable. You might want to be loved, and liked, and have friends. There are a lot of things you might want. And right now, simply notice that you want things. You don't have to do anything about it right now. Your heart will pump, your lungs will take in air, and there are many good things in life ahead of you."
(Two or three breaths.)

"And notice your thoughts, whatever they may be. You don't have to judge them right now, or change them, or fix them, or worry about them. Simply notice them, flowing through your mind. And notice how your head feels, resting on the ground. And you have wonderful new thoughts and ideas ahead of you, and good things you want, and deep feelings, and right now, all you have to do is rest."
(As many breaths as feels right.)

c.   Meditation on Wholeness

A great teacher of yoga, B.K.S. Iyengar, says that meditation is becoming aware that your body is all there at the same time. The following meditation moves from part to whole to increase self-awareness and promote a fulfilling sense of self.

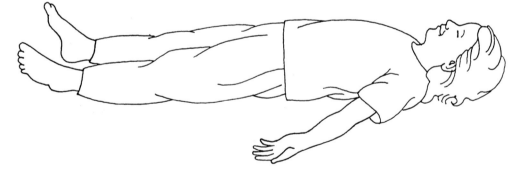

Final Relaxation

"Let's play a game to let you become more aware of your body being there. Always, there are things going on inside you that you are not aware of, but it can be surprising how much more we can notice! So, resting comfortably, notice your little left toe. Simply put your mind on your toe. Does your toe feel noticed? Maybe it does! And notice the toe next to it, and all the toes on your left foot, all there at once."

"Move your awareness to your right thumb, and back to your toes. Let your mind notice your right hand and then your left foot. You can notice both feet, very carefully. NOW, see how much of your body you can notice. Give it positive attention, so that it will feel comfortable being noticed!"

"And notice that you are all here at once. The whole thing is you and you are the whole thing. You are a whole person!"

"This is a wonderful, simple meditation that you can do lying down, sitting up, riding on a bus, waiting in line, or walking."

4.   Breathing Games

> Imagine someone tying a 50-
> pound weight to your feet and
> pushing you into a swimming
> pool. As you sink to the bottom,
> what will be your next thought?
> A new car? How is the stock
> market doing? No-o-o, I think
> your next thought will be *I have
> to breathe!*
> —Lilias Folan, *Yoga Gets Better with Age* (8)

Inhaling and exhaling in a more natural way more fully nourishes the central nervous system. The following breathing "games" are fun, playful ways to get everyone more in touch with their breathing.

a.   Breathing in Color

You can use color to connect the breath to qualities in nature like soothing water, energizing foliage, and relaxing sunlight.

"Imagine cool, calming, relaxing blue. Gently breathe in, imagining blue entering your chest, midsection, and stomach. As you release the breath, imagine that you are breathing out a yucky color, out your chest, midsection and stomach. In with the good healing blue: chest, midsection, stomach; out with the yucky color, getting rid of things you no longer need, if you ever did."
(One more breath in and out.)

"Now, imagine breathing in energizing green, full of oxygen from leaves and grass and dark green foliage. And gently exhale, and release old, dead color that you no longer need, if you ever did."

"In with good, green: chest, mid-section, stomach, and out with yucky, old stuff you can now get rid of."
(One more breath in and out.)

"And now you can imagine breathing in a gently warming yellow, warming and relaxing your chest, mid-section, and stomach, and then you can let go of old, yucky stuff you no longer need, if you ever did."

"In with beautiful, warming yellow, spreading relaxation throughout your body, and out with the stuff you no longer need, if you ever did."

"And gently let yourself breathe in, out, naturally, without having to think about it."

b.   The Special Place

The following is a "hands on" way to allow children to get in touch with their breathing in more than one way.

"And now, you will learn a simple way to take yourself to a special place. Lie still, and let your tongue gently float in your mouth. Place your hand gently on your chest and, using your breath, make your hand gently go up and down, to the rhythm of your breathing. Pretend your hand is a little boat, floating on slow, gentle waves. And it's taking you to a wonderful place. And you can decide for yourself what special place you'd like to go."
(Quiet for four breaths.)

"And let your hand glide lower down, beneath your rib-cage, and let your hand help guide your breath gently up and down. Pretend you are on your little boat, and a relaxing sun is warming you. And what a beautiful trip you are taking!"
(Five breaths.)

"And you can move your hand lower down, and place it on your stomach, and notice your hand going up and down with your breath. And now, I would like you to think of this special place this boat is taking you, and the boat is taking you closer, and closer, and closer."
(Six breaths.)

c.   Breathing Meditations

These meditations heighten bodily self-awareness. They may increase appreciation for the miracle of being alive and how resources can be shared with others. They are also a wonderful way to relax.

1)   Meditation 1

"Notice the air in the room going in the tip of your nose down into your body, and it becomes your breath. It's like magic, isn't it? Your body turns air into your breath."
(Pause for one full breath.)
"Do you notice that it feels warm where it goes in? It's still air, but it becomes something else as well, and feel the air becoming your breath."
(One full breath.)
"And as you breath in, you can feel the air becoming part of your body, your life. How does your breath feel?"
(Three full breaths.)

2)   Meditation 2

"And notice the air going out your nose, and it's warm going in and *cool* going out. How cool is that?"
(One breath.)
"Your breath inside you is precious, but the wonderful thing is how you don't hold onto it. You let it back out, and there is always more. Some very precious things in life are like that—only by not holding onto them for too long, do you get more."
(Pause for two breaths.)
"And notice the air becoming your breath, and then notice yourself letting air out of your body. And let yourself let go of any tension you are carrying, that you no longer need to hold onto, if you ever did.
(One more breath.)

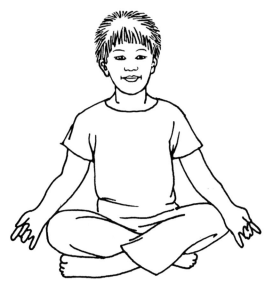

Easy Pose

5.   Balance Games

The following series of games can be tried in sequence, for balance.

a.   See the Dancer

The mind and body learn in partnership. This exercise develops the mental component of practicing yoga.

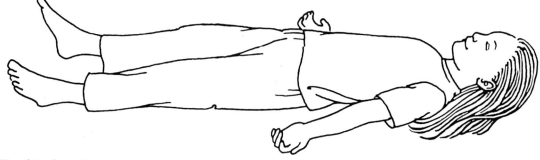

Final Relaxation

"Did you know you could practice yoga while sitting on a bus, or lying in your bed at night before sleep?"

"What about practicing Dancer Pose while lying comfortably on your back? Let's see what we can do!"

"Lie down comfortably on your back, and gently shut your eyes. See a person standing in Mountain Pose. Notice their feet spread comfortably apart. Are they barefoot? Do they have thick ankles? Notice how firmly they have those feet planted, strong and firm, like a mountain."

"Now, can you imagine this person gently lifting one foot to the back of the other knee? OK, now which foot have they lifted?"

"And now, do you see them gently wiggling the hand on the same side as the lifted up foot? Good, because now the hand is reaching around and clasping the top of the foot. The other hand floats out in front of them. Now, they gracefully bend forward from the waist and press the back leg into the hand, lifting up the leg in a nice arch behind them."

"Maybe they bend a little more and lift that leg higher! And now, they are gently coming back to earth."

"You have now practiced Dancer Pose, just while lying comfortably on your back! That is work for your brain and mind, so just take a moment and let yourself rest and see what comes."
(Pause.)

b.   Seesaw Game

Metaphor is a wonderful way to tap into the so-called "mind/body" connection that is so much a part of yoga. This little "game" taps into children's innate desire to help.

"Let's play a little balance game that you can do simply while lying back comfortably, letting your eyes rest, gently shut."

"Relax your eyelids, and let your eyeballs sort of float beneath them."

"Now, pretend that you see two children trying to play on a seesaw. One is much bigger and heavier than the other, so they are having a hard time. The bigger one comes down hard and that hurts! The smaller one stays dangling in the air, and that's no fun! Can you see the sour look on their faces?
(One breath.)

"OK, now, you are going up to the seesaw and attaching a weight on one side, to get things in balance. The children are playing now and it's even and fun, up and down, light and easy! Notice what a difference it can make to get things in balance!"
(Two breaths.)

"As you practice yoga, you can look forward to becoming more balanced in some wonderful new ways!"

c.   Tree Poem

In this exercise, the instructor will lead the class in some "poe-tree" to make Tree Pose live in their imaginations even more fully.

"OK, still resting comfortably on your back, imagine you see a forest of beautiful trees. Perhaps you notice the huge majesty of these patient, strong beings. And now, imagine that you are standing up. Without moving to get up, just pretend that you feel certain muscles working in your body, and stay nice and relaxed as you do this."

"Good work! OK, after all that exercise for your brain, let's take a break and play a game! You can all stand up and join me."

INSTRUCTOR: "Okay, we're going to learn some words we can say as we do the Tree Pose. To make it easy, first I'll say it, and then you can say it after me."
(The instructor stands on both feet, knees straight, feet about half a foot apart.)

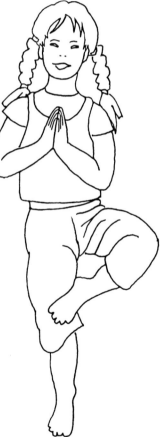

Tree Pose

Tree Poem

"Planted firmly in the ground"

    KIDS: (following the instructor) "Planted firmly in the ground"

    INSTRUCTOR: "There is a forest of breathing trees"

    KIDS: "There is a forest of breathing trees"

    (Instructor takes a big, deep breath. Kids do also.)

    INSTRUCTOR: "They grow in silence, strong and sweet"

    (Instructor lifts right foot and places it inside left calf or thigh. Kids follow suit, saying the words.)

    INSTRUCTOR: "With rain to drink and sun to eat."

    (Instructor slowly raises arms overhead, palms together, elbows back. Kids follow suit.)

    INSTRUCTOR: "From this pose, learn patience, please, And grow in balance, like the trees."

    (Kids repeat. Holding pose, instructor takes two breaths.)
"Many things reflect your worth,
Find the sky and seek the earth."

    (Instructor slowly lowers arms, lowers foot to floor. Kids do the same. Instructor repeats the exercise on the other side.)

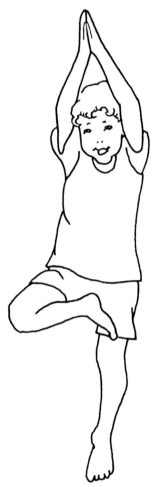

Tree Pose

6. Learning the Body

Getting in touch with your body is a wonderful way to learn about it. The focus offered by yogic relaxation can offer an opportunity for children to learn about the miraculous way the body works. Here are two examples, which children can take in as they rest with their eyes closed.

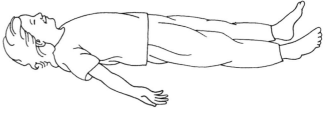

a. The Heart/Lung Connection

Final Relaxation

"Did you know that every body here is brilliant? 'Brilliant' means shining, and every body here is so smart, that intelligence shines out of you. Have you noticed? Well, I would like you to notice your body, and feel your lungs taking in oxygen."
(Two breaths.)
"And right now, your heart is pumping blood down into the lungs, where it _receives_ this wonderful oxygen that you breathe in."
(One breath.)
"Then, the heart pumps the blood back to itself, full of oxygen now, and then sends it to the rest of your body! The heart and the lungs work as a team. That is SMART, don't you think?"
(Two breaths.)

b. The Blood/Brain Barrier

"And now, notice the air coming in your nose. Your nose has little hairs that filter out the air, like a screen letting in the fresh air, but keeping out bugs."
(One breath.)
"Which is why it's a good idea to remember to breathe through your nose!"
(One breath.)
"And as your nose cleans out this air, it goes down to the lungs. The heart remembers to pump blood down to the lungs *first*, where it can get oxygen from the air. Then it pumps the blood back to itself and then all around the body. And then to the brain. And before it goes into the brain, there is something called the "blood/brain barrier," which is like another screen that filters the blood even more, to protect the brilliant and delicate brain. Did you know your body was so smart? Did you know you were so brilliant?"
(Several breaths.)

7.   Other Games

Note: Socrates says that children learn through play. Finding the "fun" side of a discipline can help children stick with it through the more difficult times.

a.   Turtle Games

There are many times in life when it is important to shift focus—from playing and having fun, to "getting serious," for example. The following games use the image of a turtle to help children learn to shift back and forth from outward to inward reality. This can develop concentration, self-awareness, self-differentiation, and can be useful in many unexpected ways.

(1)   Turtle Game 1

"Sitting comfortably, shut your eyes and imagine a turtle—in any way that you'd like...
(Two breaths)
and the turtle is moving its neck in and out, and a neck is a nice thing to have, isn't it? It can move in so many directions!
(One breath.)
And move your neck in and out, in any way that you'd like.
(One or two breaths.)
The wonderful thing about a turtle is that he can go into himself or out into the world very easily. And you can do that too, but in your own special way. So now relax and imagine the whole world outside you.
(Two breaths.)
And now point your awareness inward and imagine the whole world inside you. Inside your head and body and mind."
(Two or more breaths – whatever feels comfortable.)

(2)   Turtle Game 2

"And now, let's get in Child's Pose. Sit back on your heels and rest your head on the floor. Gently place your arms at your sides. Take a deep breath and let out a nice 'sigh' and settle into your comfortable place.
(One breath.)
And now, feel your clothes outside you, touching your body. Feel as many places as you can where your clothes touch your body.
(One breath.)

And now feel your body from inside you, touching your clothes. See how much of your body you can feel touching your clothes.
(One breath.)

Can you feel places on your body that clothes do not touch?
(One breath.)

And, in any way that you like, feel them touching each other - your clothes touching your body, and your body touching your clothes at the same time.
(One breath.)

And now ...feel the floor holding you up. Feel how firm and safe and secure it is. It is not going to drop you.
(One breath.)

Now, feel your body lying on the floor. Notice where it presses gently into the floor. Notice the feeling inside your body as it presses into the floor.
(One breath.)

And feel the whole floor, holding you up. There is a great, firm foundation beneath you. Beneath you is the great, steady earth.
(One breath.)

Again, feel your body, lying on the floor. Notice what a wonderful job it is doing, relaxing, and pressing gently against the floor.
(One breath.)

And, in any way that you would like, feel both at once—the floor holding up your body, and your body resting on the floor. Notice the place where they touch—the border—where you can feel the floor holding you up and your body resting on the floor, both at the same time.
(Two or three breaths.)

And remember the turtle, and your neck will be there whenever you need it."

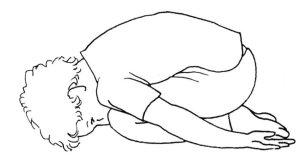

Child's Pose

b.   Flow Game

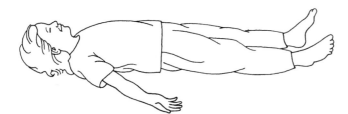

Final Relaxation

"Imagine a great flow of water—a waterfall, a river, a gentle brook, a rushing stream. Let your imagination flow with the water. Notice the flow of your breathing." (Two or three breaths.)

"Did you know that bodies of water cover 75% of the earth's surface? The average body is more than half water. It is natural to let your body and mind flow together."
(Several breaths.)

c.   Oil Can

"Pick one of your knee—it doesn't matter which on—you decide. In your imagination, pretend that a healing, lubricating oil is oozing and easing its way onto that knee joint. And now, the other knee joint as well. There is enough left over to spread its way to wherever it might be needed—the hips, the spine, shoulders, wrists, fingers, ankles, mingling and tingling its way into your beautiful, wonderful joints."

d.   Patting Yourself on the Back

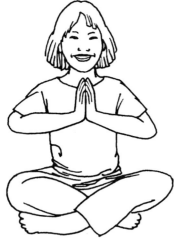

Easy Pose

"Sit in Easy Pose. You can shut your eyes comfortably and think about all the amazing things your body does for you. If you look at something, your eyes see it for you. Notice your breathing and think of three other things your body does for you."
(Two or three breaths.)

"Does everybody have three things? Imagine that you want to thank your body for these and many other things it does for you. Cup your right hand and reach around in front of your chin and gently pat behind your left shoulder. Imagine that you are thanking your body for a job well done! If you like, you can gently massage the shoulder muscles and then pat it again."

"Well done! And now, reach the left hand around and gently pat your right shoulder. Then, if you like, you can give it a little massage, and gently pat yourself on the back again. We all deserve a pat on the back sometimes."

C. Yoga in the Classroom

Yoga in the classroom provides a wonderful physical and mental break for both kids and teachers. Five minutes of stretching the muscles, deepening the breath, and clearing the mind can be just the break everyone needs to get back on task. These poses are also great to do when studying at home or at the library.

1. Yoga in Your Chair

a. Gentle Twist

"Now we are going to take a break and let our bodies stretch our minds! Make your spine straight and tall as you gently roll your shoulders back. Fill your lungs with new air by taking a deep breath in. Gently turn and put your right hand on the back of the top of your chair as you look over your left shoulder. Feel your right side stretch. Take two breaths here. Now switch sides."

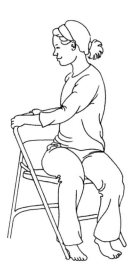

Chair Twist

b. Forward Bend

"Open your knees so that your feet are hooked on the outside of your chair. Gently allow yourself to melt forward. Extra blood is going to your brain! Take two deep breaths here and slowly come up to sitting."

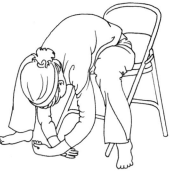

Chair Forward Bend

c. Side Stretch

"Put your right hand on the outside of your chair seat. Slowly breathe your left arm up and reach it over your head toward the right. You are a half moon shining brightly. Slowly release the arm and stretch the other side."

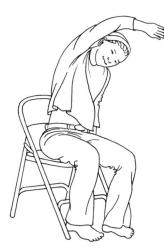

Chair Side Stretch

d. Breathing

"As you take a deep breath, raise your arms over your head and press your palms together, index fingers pointing to the sky. Exhale as you release your hands down to your side. Let's do this three times as you move with your breath. Breathe in as your hands go up, breathe out as your arms come down.

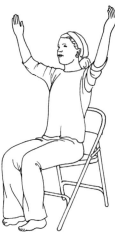

Chair Breathing

2. Yoga by Your Desk

a. Mountain Pose

"Stand next to your desk in Mountain Pose Reach your hands to the sky and stretch out your legs and arms."

b. Rooster Pose

"Now stretch up and stand on your tip toes! Remember to breathe in as your reach for the sky."

c. King Dancer

"Bend your right leg, reach around and grab your foot with your right hand. Gently kick into your right hand and feel the stretch. If you like, slowly bend forward, still hold ing your leg. Now do the left side so it gets a good stretch and new blood to the muscles."

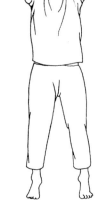

Rooster Pose

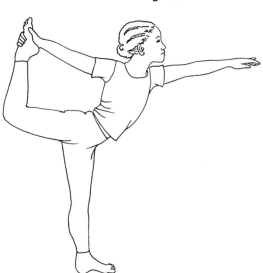

Mountain Pose

King Dancer

d. Crescent Moon

"Stand in Mountain Pose. Reach your arms up. Take your right hand and gently grasp your left wrist. Slowly pull your left arm over your head into a crescent shape. Breathe! Come back to neutral with your arms up straight. Then do the other side."

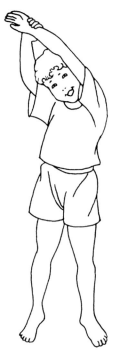

Crescent Moon

e.   Chair Pose

"We aren't ready to sit in our chairs yet, but let's take another kind of seat. Hold your arms out in front of you, and as if you are holding on to a bar, lean back. Your knees should bend as if you were sitting in a chair. Breathe into all those large muscles in your legs. Come back up to standing and shake out your legs."

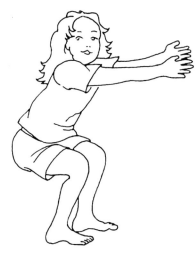

Chair Pose

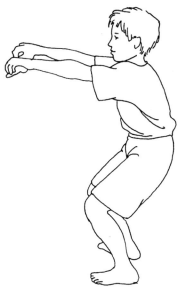

Chair Pose

Final Note:
Perhaps by introducing kids to yoga...they can remember years later...a certain something...that made them feel a certain way, not really sure what or why, but just enough to give them the idea to try yoga...and perhaps find some centering in their lives.

As St. Augustine said,
>*Since you cannot do good to all, you*
>*are to pay special attention to those*
>*who, by accidents of time, or place,*
>*or circumstance, are brought into*
>*closer connection with you.*

NAMASTE ~

Sanskrit Pronunciations*

Asana: (AHS-anna). *asana*=seat

Bow pose: *Dhanurasana* (don-your-AHS-anna). *dhanu*=bow

Bridge Pose: *Setu Bandha (*SET-too BAHN-dah*). setu*=dam, dike, or bridge *bandha*=lock

Butterfly: (Bound Angle Pose) *Baddha Konasana* (BAH-dah cone-AHS-anna). *baddha*=bound; *kona*=angle

Chair Pose: *Utkatasana* (OOT-kah-TAHS-anna*). Utkata*=powerful, fierce

Child's Pose: *Balasana* (bah-LAHS-anna). *Bala*=child

Cobra Pose: *Bhujangasana* (boo-jang-GAHS-anna). *Bhujanga*=serpent, snake

Downward-Facing Dog. *Adho Mukha Svanasana (AH-doh MOO-kah shvah-NAHS-anna). adho*=downward; *mukha*=face; *svana*=dog

Eagle Pose: *Garudasana* (gah-rue-DAHS-anna)

Fish Pose: *Matysasana (*mot-see-AHS-anna*). matsya*=fish

Forward Bend (standing): *Uttanasana* (OOT-tan-AHS-ahna*). utt*=intense; *tan*-to stretch or extend

Half Moon Pose: Ardha Chandrasana (are-dah chan-DRAHS-anna). Ardha=half; *candra*=glittering, shining, having the brilliancy or hue of light (said of the gods); usually translated as "moon"

Half Shoulderstand: Ardha Sarvangasana (ARE-dah sar-van-GAHS-anna)

King Dancer or Lord of the Dance Pose. *Natarajasana (not-ah-raj-AHS-anna). Nata*=actor, dancer, mime *raja*=king

Legs-Up-the-Wall Pose: *Viparita Karani* (vip-par-ee-tah car-AHN-ee*)* Viparita=turned around, reversed, inverted karani=doing, making, action

Mountain Pose: Tadasana *(tah-DAHS-anna).* tada=mountain

Prayer Pose: *Anjali Mudra* (Salutation Seal). *Anjali*=a gesture of reverence, salutation *mudra*=seal (The gesture "seals" energy in the body)

Pretzel Pose or Half Lord of the Fishes Pose: *Ardha Matsyendrasana* (ARE-dah MOT-see-en-DRAHS-anna). *ardha*=half**.** *Matsyendra*=king of the fish; *matsya*=fish; *indra*=ruler

Rocket Pose: (Side-Angle Pose) *Parsvakonasana* (parsh-vah-cone-AHS-anna) *Parsva*=side; *kona*=angle

Rainbow Pose: Vasisthasana (vah-sish-TAHS-anna). *Vasistha*=literally means "most excellent, best, richest."

Savasana: (shah-VAHS-anna) *sava*=corpse

Tree Pose: *Vrksasana* (vrik-SHAHS-anna). *vrksa*=tree

Upward-Facing Dog: *Urdhva Mukha Svanasana* (ERD-vah MOO-kah shvon-AHS-anna). *urdhva mukha*=face upward; *urdhva*=upward; *mukha*=face; *svana*=dog

Warrior 1, 2, and 3: *Virabhadrasana* 1, 2, and 3 (veer-ah-bah-DRAHS-anna)

* Special Thanks to Yoga Journal. More information available at: http://www.yogajournal.com/poses/index.cfm?ctsrc=channel

References

(1) Mohan, A.G. *Yoga for Body, Breath, and Mind*. Boston: Shambhala. 2002.

(2) Ornish, Dean. *Dr. Dean Ornish's Program for Reversing Heart Disease: The Only System Scientifically Proven to Reverse Heart Disease Without Drugs or Surgery*. New York: Random House. 1990.

(3) Benson, Herbert. *The Relaxation Response*. New York: HarperTorch. 1976.

(4) Farhi, Donna. *Yoga Mind, Body & Spirit: A Return to Wholeness*. New York: Henry Holt and Company. 2000.

(5) Devi, Nischala Joy. *The Healing Path of Yoga*. New York: Three Rivers Press. 2000.

(6) Iyengar, B.K.S. *Yoga: The Path of Holistic Health*. New York: Dorling Kindersley. 2001.

(7) Payne, Larry, and Richard Usatine. *Yoga Rx*. New York: Random House. 2002.

(8) Folan, Lilias. *Yoga Gets Better With Age*. Rodale Press. 2005.

Printed in the United States
219728BV00002B/9/A